Praise for **Declarative Language Handbook**

"When I heard that Linda Murphy was writing "Declarative Language Handbook", a hallmark of RDI, I knew that our Autism and Communication worlds were about to influenced by the cutting edge thinking of a truly remarkable expert in the field. What I wasn't prepared for were the crisp, practical, useful guidelines that will make this the most important book on the shelf of clinicians and parents dealing with autism. The Declarative Language Handbook outlines specific strategies in a fresh, hands-on and real-world way. I recommend this book without reservation."

-Rachelle K. Sheely PhD
President & Co-Founder of RDIConnect

"As a seasoned clinician, I found that when I changed my language from imperative to declarative, I started to notice new competencies of children. I am continually amazed at how simple (but difficult!) changes in my language can be so powerful and bring about incredible changes in a short time. We are so fortunate to have Linda explain the principles of Declarative Language in a book. Over the years, I have applied parts of this approach with Linda's gentle guidance as a colleague. Yet, to have it all explained in one place, with excellent examples and practice opportunities, is so valuable. Thank you Linda for putting all the resources in one place, and, with this help, onward with my journey!"

-Martha Bargmann MS, CCC-SLP
Speech Language Pathologist at Massachusetts General Hospital *for* Children

"I am so happy to see a book dedicated to declarative language. The shift to increased student agency and teachers as coaches is dependent on a new kind of language in the classroom. Declarative language elevates teaching to that new level."
                        -Melissa Andrichak MAT, First Grade Teacher

"Finally! An easy to read book that meets parents and educators 'in the trenches' with information and strategies that help our kids learn critical thinking, social problem solving and executive functioning skills. This book is proof of how making small shifts in our language can have far reaching results for our kids in the areas of social communication, problem solving and self regulation!"
        -Beckham Linton MA, CCC-SLP, Social Learning Consultant /Coach
                                Heartland Social Learning Center LLC

"The content is organized in a way that I found it very user friendly and generous, even providing tips for skipping chapters! The writing style flows with kindness and meaning. The content goes beyond "technical." It talks about relating to others with deep respect, since we are all different from each other. It inspires us beyond being a better clinician, but to be better as humans! I already find myself rethinking how I can present my comments and requests in a more declarative/reflective way, with my clients, kids, husband, and during staff meetings at work.

I have been trying to use declarative language since I first heard about it, but this book brings it to a new level of understanding and support, and makes it easier to apply. It has already saved me from a few confrontations! Every time I use declarative language and it works, I think to myself: *Thank you Linda!*"
        -Vania Machado MS, CCC-SLP, Speech Language Pathologist
        Early Intervention through Elementary School, Clinical Supervisor

"Linda beautifully describes a communication style that can influence how children perceive their environment, which in turn can increase their level of engagement in the world around them. Declarative language, as described in this handbook, is a relationship-based approach to help children foster competence and confidence as communicators. If you're a self-reflective person, you will enjoy this read! "

-Hillary L. Perron, OTR/L, Occupational Therapist

"A wonderful guide for using declarative language when speaking with children who have social learning challenges. As an adult diagnosed with Asperger's Syndrome, I understand the importance of helping children with social learning challenges become more confident with conversations and cope with perfectionism. The book explains perfectly how changing our language from imperative to declarative can make a world of difference when engaging in conversation with children."

-Carla M.

"This book is practical and so user friendly. Each chapter is full of examples and stories that make it real. It's great to now be able to offer families and providers a comprehensive resource on declarative language. When I consult to schools, this is a tool I always discuss - and now I can offer them far more information. Thanks for finding the time to share your passion - to educate the world of the power of declarative language - to give people a step by step approach with many examples and tools to make the shift to declarative language."

-Deirdre Mulcahy Patch MS, CCC-SLP
Feeding Therapist/Speech Language Pathologist

Declarative Language Handbook

Using a Thoughtful Language Style to Help Kids
with Social Learning Challenges Feel Competent,
Connected, and Understood

Linda K. Murphy MS, CCC-SLP

First paperback edition February 2020

Book design by Brent Spears

ISBN 978-1-7345162-0-3 (paperback)
ISBN 978-1-7345162-1-0 (ebook)

Library of Congress Control Number: 2020901193

www.declarativelanguage.com

DEDICATION

For Noah, Ben, Regina and Jason. Thank you for always believing in my work and pushing me to reach as high as I can.

Contents

PART 4: PACING AND TROUBLESHOOTING

PART 5: PRACTICE

PART 6: TRACKING PROGRESS AND RESEARCH

PART 7: FINAL WORDS

ACKNOWLEDGEMENTS

I'd like to express heartfelt gratitude to Dr. Steven E. Gutstein, Dr. Rachelle K. Sheely, and the RDI® Community for introducing me to a different way of teaching kids with social communication challenges. Their visionary approach to ASD and other developmental difficulties has positively impacted and influenced me as a clinician in ways too numerous to count. Putting their ideas into practice over the past 13 years has given me the experience and confidence to now share some of this knowledge with others.

I'd also like to thank Michelle Garcia Winner, Dr. Pamela Crooke, and the Social Thinking® Community. The publishing of my first book, *Social Thinking and Me*, which I co-authored with Michelle, helped me gain the confidence and desire to do this again. As leaders in the field, Michelle and Pam show me every day that changing the world is possible.

I am eternally grateful to all the families I have worked with over the years. You have shown me what a difference a positive communication style can make. Thank you especially to the families who allowed me to share their stories in this book.

I am thankful to our team at Peer Projects Therapy From the Heart. You share my vision for kids with social learning challenges and fulfill this important work every day.

Last but certainly not least, I am thankful to Rob, Freddie and Desmond for always supporting my work and encouraging me to write this book.

PART I

INTRODUCTION

Why Are We Here?

I recently read that the most important thing we can give to each other these days is time. Thank you for giving me your time and attention right now. I will do my best to not take it for granted and will get right to the point of why we are here and what I want you to learn.

I have been talking about and advocating for the use of declarative language since I first learned about it in 2007 while training to become a Relationship Development Intervention® (RDI) Consultant. RDI is a developmental treatment approach founded by Dr. Steven E. Gutstein and Dr. Rachelle K. Sheely. By training parents, RDI helps kids with social learning challenges develop social competence and social connection. These areas are the most important to me as a clinician. Declarative language immediately became one of the most important tools in my toolbox when guiding social learning. I also quickly came to believe that this understated tool should be in every educator and caregiver's toolbox.

As I started regularly using declarative language with my clients, and later on with my own kids, I realized how empowering and refreshing the use of this tool is. An official Declarative Language Handbook for how to use this speaking style with kids who have social learning challenges has not yet been published, so I decided it was time to create one.

My goal in writing this book is to help everyone understand the power of declarative language and understand that its benefits are far-reaching and important. My goal is also to help parents, teachers, caregivers, and all those who care about someone with social learning challenges, realize that they can use it immediately and effectively. Anyone reading this book can learn how to speak in a declarative way. And by doing so, you will all become aware that what you say and how you say it matters. Paying attention to our own speaking style can make the difference between a child shutting down and a child opening themselves up to learning.

I am eager to get on with this teaching, to say the least! But first, let's back up to start on the same page.

I think most people agree the following areas are difficult for individuals with social learning challenges: seeing the big picture, being flexible, managing impulses, taking the perspective of others, problem solving in real time, and reading nonverbal communication. For some kids, learning how to connect with others through the sharing of memories, making plans for the near and distant future, and expressing emotions can also be a challenge.

These are all big areas to consider and big areas to target. They are also areas that are constantly intertwined into every interaction and social opportunity that we have in life. Wouldn't it be great if there was a way that we could support growth in these areas that was also woven into everyday interactions and social opportunities? And even better—what if it was something that a parent or caregiver could use in the moment, to guide kids or adults towards improved social learning?

That is what this book is about. It's to help you, the person who cares deeply about someone with social learning challenges, know how to use these everyday incidental moments to teach and guide social learning. You might be a therapist or a teacher, or you might be a parent, grandparent, or babysitter. The point of this book is to help you feel equipped to make a difference simply by being mindful of your own communication and speaking style, no matter what your relationship to the child happens to be.

Here are some example moments where social learning can happen. They may seem small, but small moments add up over time.

Moments at home: The cat needs to be fed. You are having breakfast with your child. The trash needs to be taken out. Packing lunches for school. It's recycling day tomorrow and you need to get it all to the curb! Oh no… yard work again. Water spilled. You think it would be fun to make popcorn. Gotta make that peanut butter and jelly sandwich for snack time. Sorting socks that just came out of the dryer.

Moments in school: Letting the kids know it's almost time for recess. Someone didn't hang up their coat. Test time! A pencil broke. Recycling time again and you need helpers. Kids need to take out their pencils and books for math. Did a box of markers just spill?

As a busy individual, you may be quick to tell kids what they need to do, or even do it yourself. However, life could be better if you take some of these moments and instead carve opportunities for kids to feel empowered, useful, and connected. This book is not about getting kids to do chores or do tasks though. Rather, it is about creating opportunities for them to solve problems and feel empowered themselves. It's a whole different ballgame when kids feel empowered and useful, and know they are competent.

This book is about helping kids feel more and more competent over time, as they solve bigger and more complex problems—while being guided by the language you use with them. They learn and discover what to do versus being *told* what to do (which can lead to all sorts of resistance and power struggles). When kids feel competent, they become happier kids, kids who are more open to learning, and kids who invite future learning challenges. Isn't this what we all want?

When kids feel competent, they become happier kids, kids who are more open to learning, and kids who invite future learning challenges.

The language style you are about to learn will also address a few very important areas. It will help you move away from power struggles and instead create positive connections with kids more naturally. It will help kids feel better as you validate how they are feeling while also guiding them towards more mature responses and decisions in response to their feelings. It will help kids become better able to know who they are as individuals, or in other words, increase their self-awareness. This in turn will lead to them being better able to self-advocate in both the near and far future. This is what is most important. We want our kids to be able to advocate for what they need in ways that others will understand and respond to positively.

The flip side to areas of challenge… areas of growth! Specific areas in relation to social learning challenges that will grow with the help of declarative language will be discussed in upcoming chapters. These include observation, episodic memory, tolerating, accepting and embracing different opinions, feeling okay making mistakes, and thinking in alternatives.

Chapter 1: Why Are We Here?

I often remember one thing that Dr. Steven Gutstein said during my RDI training that helped change my mindset. He said, "We need to move from *get* to *give*. We want to get rid of the *get*." I go back to his words often when I'm with kids. What he meant was that I needed to shift away from trying to "get" kids or adults with social learning challenges to do something, and instead get better at "giving." As we give them more from the heart—more information, more understanding, more compassion, more patience—it is amazing to see what they will give back. But it has to start with us.

We can help kids be open to guidance in the moment. We can help them engage in opportunities where they can contribute in meaningful ways. We can help them feel comfort and enjoyment when learning new things. And we can help them make positive and lasting social connections with others. We can do all these things once we stop to think about what we say and how we say it. That is what this book is about.

A note about how to use this book

There is a lot of information in the pages ahead. If you are interested in the rationale of why to use declarative language as well as how to do it, I suggest you read the chapters in order. Part 2 will be of special interest to you because in these chapters I explain in detail different areas important for social learning and social competence. This explanation will lay the groundwork for understanding the power of declarative language.

But if you are eager to get started using declarative language and want to know how best to construct declarative statements, you should read Chapter 2 and then feel free to jump ahead to Parts 3 and 4. That is where I get into the mechanics of this speaking style, the importance of pacing, and troubleshooting tips. You can come back to the interesting information in Part 2 when you feel ready for it.

Part 5 provides discrete practice opportunities using practice sets, which will help you feel confident that you now know what you are doing!

Part 6 discusses the important topic of tracking progress to tell if declarative language is working and the research behind this speaking style's effectiveness in supporting social learning.

I end the handbook with a vision for the future and an invitation!

CHAPTER 2:

What You Need to Know to Get Started Right Away

It is best to start with the basics, which means we must go back to grammar class where you probably at some point learned about different sentence types. Hopefully my fourth-grade teacher, Miss Cox, would be proud that I am tackling this topic now.

Let's start with imperative language. An imperative is a question or sentence that demands a response. It might be a verbal response or an action. Imperative responses are correct or incorrect. You either answer the question right or you don't, or you perform the stated action correctly or you don't. It's black and white. Here are some examples:

Get in line.
Say hello to Grandma.
Look at me.
What did I say?
What color is your shirt?

All these imperatives have "correct" actions to perform. You either get in line or you don't. You say hello to Grandma or you don't, etc. In the world of social learning challenges, people often (and unfortunately) think first in terms of behavior. When a child doesn't do the correct action within a few seconds, this is labeled "noncompliance." What a negative word!

But here's the thing… demands can trigger, or activate, the fight/flight/freeze response. Whether real or not, the brain may interpret a demand as a threat. When this happens, the lower brain goes into a defensive or offensive state. For kids with social learning challenges, here is what that may look like:

Get in line. → Fight responses: yelling, throwing, kicking, hitting, swearing, arguing, protesting, talking back, sarcastic comment. Fight responses can be big, or they can be small.

Say hello to Grandma. → Flight responses: crawling under a table, bolting, changing the subject, saying "no" or "I don't want to." Flight responses can also be big or subtle in nature.

Look at me. → Freeze responses: not answering at all, shutting of eyes, putting the head down, seeming to "ignore" the other person. Freeze responses can be incorrectly interpreted as not caring.

Freeze responses can be incorrectly interpreted as not caring.

Remember this: you may perceive kids having one of the behaviors listed above as deliberately misbehaving, but often this is a fight, flight, or freeze response to a perceived threat, which is the demand in the moment. Imperative language places a demand on kids.

If we could change up our language so that we could teach without activating the fight/flight/freeze response, wouldn't that seem like a smart thing to do? Imagine teaching kids what we want them to learn, in a way that supports them to stay positively connected and engaged while they learn. Lower the perceived threat, increase the warmth and connection, and we all feel better.

We can do this with declarative language.

Declarative language is a comment or a statement. It is that simple. Usually it is a statement that observes. For example, it may observe events in the environment, including people, actions, and changes. It can also narrate an internal event, such as thoughts, feelings, predictions, opinions, observations, or problem-solving dialogue. It can be as simple or as complex as you'd like it to be. When using declarative language with kids with learning challenges, it will be very important to keep this in mind: Match your language complexity to the language level of the learner. In other words, speak at a level they will most likely understand.

Declarative language naturally provides opportunity for social learning across the areas of seeing the big picture, reading nonverbal communication, problem solving, perspective taking, and self-advocating.

Here is how you would turn the above imperatives into declarative statements.

Get in line. could become *I notice it's time for lunch.* or *The kids are getting ready to go into school.*

These declarative statements invite a child to look up and observe their surrounding environment. Then, once they see the contextual clues that you see (e.g., a line forming by the door), they can determine what to do next on their own: get in line. When we simply say, "Get in line," we rob them of the opportunity to see the big picture and figure out what to do on their own.

Say hello to Grandma. Grandma has arrived and greeting her is a nice thing to do right? But what if we said, *Oh look! Grandma is here!* without further instruction. This tips off the child that there has been a change in their environment, while also leaving space for them to decide how to respond to this change. Perhaps they will say hello,

11

but they also might run over to give her a hug, they might wave from where they are playing, or they might say, "Hey Grandma!" All are fine, acceptable options. The declarative statement has created space for the child to respond to Grandma's arrival in their own unique way. And because it will be spontaneous and from the heart, I'm sure Grandma will love it.

What color is your shirt? We may be asking this because we're quizzing if the child knows their colors, or perhaps to start a conversation. Either way, there are better ways to get at what's important. What if you said something like, *Hey! We have the same color shirt. I like red too.* In that moment, you are giving the child an authentic reason to notice you and your shirt, and to learn something about you. (You like the color red.) Small moments such as these help us get to know each other and over time, care about each other too. We can thoughtfully use these moments as opportunities to show a child what we have in common, what may be different about us, and that we care about them. Alternatively, if you are quizzing to help the child learn about colors, realize that quizzing and teaching are not the same thing. When we quiz, kids feel the pressure. They may also memorize the answer and say it back without necessarily understanding the concept you are teaching. In contrast, when commenting on the topic (e.g., the color of our shirts), this teaches the color in a meaningful, socially driven context. It also immediately helps the concept generalize – i.e., we are both wearing red shirts, even though the "reds" may be slightly different. This natural way of learning feels better to everyone involved.

The next two examples really get at the heart of some of the most important benefits of declarative language. Demands can make kids feel inadequate. But declarative language empowers them to feel competent, understand the world better, develop self-awareness, and self-advocate.

Demands can make kids feel inadequate. But declarative language empowers them to feel competent, understand the world better, develop self-awareness, and self-advocate.

Look at me. When we say this, we are demanding attention. We are telling a child very directly to look at us. But why? We don't say. Also, we are not being sensitive to the fact that for some kids with social learning challenges, it can be very hard to look and listen at the same time. Instead, what if we use a statement to give information about the social context and to teach the importance of observation such as, *I'm worried you might miss something important if you don't look.* In that moment, you are not demanding eye contact. Rather, you are inviting them to observe because it is important. You are communicating that you care about their learning.

When a phrase like this is followed by a silent pause, the child will often look on their own. Then you can show them what it is you want them to see. They will be ready to take it in because you have allowed them time to become ready for new information. In contrast, if we make them look before they are ready, this can lead to feelings of stress. And stress impedes learning.

What did I say? Okay, so I admit I'm guilty of asking this question to my own children when I feel like they are not listening. But it is one that I work to handle differently. For kids with language difficulties, who may struggle with auditory memory, comprehension, or distractibility, this question can be hard to answer, and as result, shaming. For example, if we ask, *What did I say?* and the child can't answer, the child feels bad but so do we.

Fortunately, there is a better way! What if instead we say, *I'm wondering if you heard what I said,* or *I'm not sure you heard me,* or even *I want to make sure we are on the same page. It will help me if I know that you heard me.* Then any of these statements, paired with a deliberate and considerate pause, can result in a response that leads to self-advocacy. For example, maybe the child who struggles with remembering language will say, "I heard you but I forgot." Or the child with comprehension challenges will say, "I heard you but I didn't understand," Or the distracted child may say, "I didn't hear you because of the fan." Each of these responses will then in turn lead to a compassionate and helpful response from us. In the process, it helps us understand that child's learning style (strengths and weaknesses) a little bit more. It creates a situation in which a child can feel empowered to get the help they need, rather than shamed by their vulnerabilities.

Declarative language creates a situation in which a child can feel empowered to get the help they need, rather than shamed by their vulnerabilities.

In the event that a child does not yet have the language or self-awareness to self-advocate, you can guide this learning based on your own experiences with that child: *I'm thinking maybe it was hard for you to hear me with the fan going,* or *I think you heard me but maybe you forgot,* or even *I think there may have been a new word in there. Maybe you didn't understand what I said.* All of these are so much better than the awful silence you get when you ask a child, "What did I say?" and they can't answer.

Here is the sad truth. People often use imperative language with kids who have social learning or other language learning challenges. They make the incorrect assumption that a child will not understand a declarative statement or that the child is not at a level where they could benefit from it. This is not true. What is important to think about is not the style of language you are using (imperative over declarative) but rather the complexity. You can make a simple declarative statement that is understandable, when paired with other scaffolds. (We'll get to these in Chapter 11.) Kids with less developed language may need simpler language, and at times most certainly need clear imperatives, but they do not need imperatives ALL the time. If we want kids to feel connected and develop both social connection and joint attention, we must start with our own communication. We must use a speaking style that fosters this type of communication. Imperative language does not foster social connection or social inter-action. Declarative statements do.

I want to end this chapter with two personal examples of when I have been moved by the power of declarative language. When I first began my training as an RDI Consultant, I was working with a three-year-old girl, Eliza. You will hear more stories of her through-out this book. Interactions with her provided me opportunity for my first attempts using declarative language. I clearly remember working with Eliza on a wooden doll dress-up set one day. As she placed a small cloth around the doll's neck, I made the declarative statement, *Hmm... I wonder what that could be.* In my head, I was thinking it looked like a necktie, and expected Eliza to say that too. But after a short pause while Eliza thought about my statement, she responded, "It's a scarf!" She was right, it did also look like a scarf! I was blown away in that moment, not by her response, but by my discovery. Because I left the door open for Eliza to think and respond in her own unique way, her idea—which was different than mine—shone through. I responded with genuine delight, "Yes it does look like a scarf! I was thinking it was a necktie!" As a result of declarative language, we were both provided with an opportunity to learn about perspective (we each viewed the cloth differently) and alternative thinking (realization that the cloth could be thought about in different ways). This moment has always stuck with me because it made me realize I was going to learn a lot from declarative language.

Because I left the door open for Eliza to think and respond in her own unique way, her idea—which was different from mine—shone through.

The second example came several years later after I started working with 21-year-old Christopher and his mother, Judy. Judy contacted me because, although she felt very close to her son, his communication was limited. They had their shared routines and connections, but she wanted to help him better express himself to both herself and to others. Christopher's father had passed away when he was 9. Christopher was a concrete learner who had been in a residential school since he was 12 years old because, as a single mother, Judy felt she could not keep him safe when he began unlocking the front door and leaving the house in the middle of the night. Christopher continued to come home from the school every weekend, and they had phone calls during the week, but Judy shared that it was difficult to start a conversation with him or establish deeper communication.

Due to Christopher's perceived learning potential, people usually used imperative language with him. They asked him questions, gave him directions, and so on. When we started working together, the first thing I guided Judy to practice was using declarative statements. Judy learned to stop asking questions, and instead make comments about what they were doing together.

Judy and Christopher used to make "pals" together. These were creations of Christopher's beloved cartoon characters made out of

16

felt. I joined them in this activity one day, and Judy and I used guiding statements to help Christopher know what to do. Examples included: *Let's put glue here,* or *I remember your mom smudged the glue to spread it,* and *Let's flip this over together... I'll take this side.* Christopher stayed engaged throughout, asking follow-up questions like "What's smudge mean?", taking ownership of his role, spontaneously orienting his body toward the activity, and leaning in when he had a job to do. This 21-year-old man, though quiet, stayed engaged as our language shifted to a positive style that provided him with information, guided him as to what to do, and never once placed a demand on him to do or say something. Years later, Christopher is now a very chatty guy who shares his thoughts often. You will hear more stories about him later in this book too. Today Judy and I think back to the days when he couldn't share as much as he can now, and we are in awe of the power of declarative language.

I also want to be clear in saying that declarative language does not fix language challenges outright, and changes do not happen overnight. The changes in communication that I'm describing happen at a different pace for everyone. But for all learners, it helps in one important way. Consistent use of declarative language creates a communicative landscape that is positive and inviting for kids with social learning challenges. It leaves space for kids to be themselves, feel comfortable, and let their guard down. Over time, this welcoming backdrop helps kids stay open to learning and stay connected to us, especially as things get challenging. This is what is most important and will serve kids in the long term, through the ups and downs of learning.

There is more to come in Chapter 8 about the specific nuts and bolts of declarative statements, and how to construct declarative statements in varied ways. But first, we will discuss the areas of social learning that declarative language helps to develop.

PART 2:

GETTING TO THE GOOD STUFF–SOCIAL LEARNING AREAS FOSTERED BY DECLARATIVE LANGUAGE

CHAPTER 3:
Moving Beyond Eye Contact

For as long as I can remember, people have been telling kids with autism to "look at me" or demanding eye contact. When I was training to become an RDI Consultant, however, I learned there is a completely different way to think about eye contact, and one that immediately felt so much better to me. But let me back up and define the idea of "making eye contact." When demanded, eye contact is positioned as a rote skill. It is discrete. The child looks and they're done. When we communicate though, there is so much more going on when a person "looks." And there is a much better term for what is actually happening: visual referencing.

Visual referencing refers to the process of using our sense of sight to gain information: we are referencing our surroundings to learn more. We may be gaining information about our immediate environment, or we may be gaining information about the people we are with—our communication partners. Here is an example. Imagine are walking down the street late at night. You bet you are going visually reference the environment to ensure you are safe! Or how about crossing the street? Of course you are going to look to the left and then to the right, and maybe back again, to determine whether it is safe to cross. You are noticing the context, interpreting what you see, and taking action based on this information. Another example: imagine you go to a party. As you enter, you visually reference the space to figure out the lay of the land (Where's the food? Where are the drinks? Where are the bathrooms?) and to find someone that will anchor you (Do I see anyone I know? Who can I talk to?).

With communication partners, we must visually reference all the time. For example, imagine you are telling a friend about your weekend. You visually check in often to see if they are listening, to see if they understand what you are saying, and to see if they are even interested! They will communicate all of these things through their facial expressions and other nonverbal communication. But you need to look to figure this out.

Here's the bottom line: looking just by itself (or "eye contact") is not nearly enough to get at the dynamic nature of communication. Rather, we must help our kids with social learning challenges become better at visually referencing.

Here's the bottom line: looking just by itself (or "eye contact") is not nearly enough to get at the dynamic nature of communication. Rather, we must help our kids with social learning challenges become better at visually referencing.

There are a few elements to keep in mind with regards to visual referencing. First, just because kids are looking up doesn't mean they will notice what is socially meaningful in that moment. Thus, once we help kids feel comfortable looking, we must guide them as to *what* to notice. Second, we want to help kids visually reference more often. A lot of kids with social learning challenges tend to keep their heads down. It may be because they are working hard on listening, and it can be hard to look and listen at the same time. But it also may be because they are used to others telling them what to do, or used to being prompted. If we want to guide kids toward independence, we want to help them feel comfortable looking more often. We also want to help them understand this is important. Lastly, once kids know what to observe, and are in fact looking more often, we will most likely need to help them derive meaning from what they are seeing. Kids with social learning challenges do not necessarily know right away how to decode nonverbal or contextual information. It will be our job to help them understand what they are seeing.

Visual referencing is a dynamic skill, important for communicative success and independence. It is imperative that those teaching kids with social learning challenges understand the difference between eye contact and visual referencing, so that the latter skill can develop.

Now that you understand the difference, here is the great news! Declarative language naturally guides kids to visually reference. It gets at the heart of this skill by helping kids to (1) know what to observe, (2) feel comfortable observing more often, and (3) derive meaning from what they are seeing. Declarative language gives individuals in the moment teaching, practice, and support across each of these areas.

Here are several example declarative statements that support visual referencing, along with their imperative counterparts (that you used to use, but are now working hard to change, right?).

Your body is on top of the pieces! This is a personal example with my son, Freddie, who was seven at the time. I have it on video and show it to others often as it illustrates the simple but dynamic nature of visual referencing. I was gearing up to play a game with both of my sons, but Freddie was sitting on top of everything. He did not realize this and did not notice how his body impacted the rest of us. As I made this declarative statement, he did not respond right away. But after a few seconds, he said, "Huh?" and looked up from the toy he was holding. He looked at the floor around him, saw that he was in fact sitting on top of everything, and then moved his body back. In this one 30-second clip, he visually references his surroundings (takes in the big picture), and moves back (problem solving) in a way that helps others (perspective taking). In contrast, if I had simply said, "Move back Freddie," he would have followed the direction, but it is unlikely he would have visually referenced the context in the same way, and the problem solving would have been mine, not his.

You're stepping on your shirt. This is another personal example and a video clip that I share often for the same reason. What can I say? My kids are working on body awareness! In this example, my younger son, Desmond, was putting away his laundry... while dancing! He did not notice that a clean shirt had fallen to the floor and was under his feet. I made the statement above, and after a couple of seconds he paused, said "Huh?" and then looked to the floor. He noticed the shirt, picked it up, and continued with his chore. A "Huh?" is a good indicator that you are onto great things: the child has just realized there is a problem to solve. In my video clip, we can see Desmond visually reference his surroundings (see the big picture), pause his dance routine (self-regulate), and then made a great choice in picking it up (problem solve). Again, if I had simply used an imperative: "Get off that shirt," all those beautiful and nuanced moments of social learning would have been lost.

If I had simply used an imperative: "Get off that shirt," all those beautiful and nuanced moments of social learning would have been lost.

Last example for now.

I wonder what the other kids are doing. Imagine you are encouraging a child with social learning challenges to play with other kids on the playground. But that child is not sure how to join or seems to prefer doing their own thing. If you can help that child feel at ease simply observing the other kids without pressure to join just yet, it is a comfortable way to begin the process of joining. Here is what you can do: stand alongside that child and make the declarative statement *I wonder what the other kids are doing.* The child won't feel pressure to do anything specific that would create worry or anxiety and has space to simply scan the playground with you.

You can guide further as needed. Once you see the child look up, guide their observation toward the right place with another declarative statement, *I see them right over by the sandbox.* You can then take the opportunity to help the child understand what they are seeing. *It looks like they are playing at the sandbox. I can see them filling up a dump truck with sand and pouring it into a bucket.* You are guiding the child to visually reference, helping them know where to look, and then helping them understand or derive meaning from what they are seeing, all using declarative statements.

You may even take it a step further and make a simple invitation such as, *I wonder if you'd like to join them...* No pressure, just a simple invitation, which the child could accept, but if not, that is okay too.

The child may join next time because they'll now understand what they are seeing and feel more comfortable approaching as a result.

This important in the moment teaching would be lost if you used an imperative, *Go play with the other kids*, or if you asked, *What are the other kids doing?* The imperative statement places a demand on the child which may cause stress, and the question is a big one that our kids with social learning challenges may not be able to answer. Either could activate a fight/flight/freeze response. In contrast, declarative statements will thoughtfully guide, generate curiosity and wonder about peers, and provide opportunity for the child with social learning challenges to consider a new play opportunity.

As we move onto other areas of social learning, remember to think beyond eye contact. Use declarative language to foster visual referencing instead. Most importantly, be sure to pause after each statement to allow time for the child to process what you have said, and have their own "aha!" moment. (Or the case of my kids, "Huh?") Take pride as you start to notice how the child begins to look up spontaneously, noticing and figuring things out their own.

CHAPTER 4:
Using Episodic Memory for Problem Solving

In this chapter I will discuss episodic memory. There are many different types of memory, but I want to teach you about episodic memory because it is vital for social competence. Episodic memory is what we use to recall memories or past experiences that are relevant in the here and now. Whenever we are in a new situation, our brain automatically goes through its internal Rolodex of files to find a match. Although this is largely an unconscious process, we often think, "Where have I been in the past that reminds me of this place?" Or "When have I been in a situation like this in the past and what did I do then?" Our minds are constantly searching for matches and patterns so that we know what to do in the moment. If you consider yourself socially competent, chances are your episodic memory is strong. Every time you enter a novel context or situation, you don't freak out because you can figure out what to do based on your past experiences.

Episodic memory is what we use to recall memories or past experiences that are relevant in the here and now.

Now think of the flip side. If your episodic memory is weak, each and every novel situation, interaction, and environment would feel brand new. You wouldn't be able to recall and use knowledge from similar, past experiences. As a result, you would feel stuck when faced with a new or even slightly new problem, situation, or communication partner. You may even feel frightened, depending how dynamic the context was.

Here are two examples.

When I was in college, I backpacked around Europe with my friend Maria. We went to Prague in what was then Czechoslovakia. I vividly remember going into a grocery store. So many things were different. The language was different, the food was different, and the aisles were narrower than the ones I was used to in big American grocery stores. Now if I focused on the differences, I'm sure I would've felt stuck or even scared. However, because I have intact episodic memory, my brain naturally guided me to notice the similarities. Yes, there were many differences, but overall what I was experiencing matched a template in my brain called "grocery store." There were still aisles, still food on shelves, still baskets to carry, and a cashier whom we paid when we were done. So many things were different, but Maria and I could figure out what to do because we knew how grocery stores worked. We were (mostly!) socially competent in this environment that was foreign to us. It is really amazing to consider!

Here is another example. Recently we took a family trip to Legoland in Florida. Due to a snowstorm back home, our flight got canceled and the airline couldn't get us home for three days. There are, of course, worse things that could happen than being stuck in Florida in the middle of winter! But from a practicality standpoint, we had to figure out what to do and where to stay. We had been at Legoland for three nights, and to stay there longer (as much as we loved it) would be financially prohibitive. As I flipped through my own episodic memory in search of a good match to this problem, I recalled that my uncle lives in Florida, only two hours from Legoland. We made the calls, he had extra room, and the decision was made to stay with him and my aunt for a few days. We found a reasonable and even enjoyable solution without too much worry, because my episodic memory works well. In contrast, if my episodic memory had not been as strong, we could've ended up paying a lot more money than we had budgeted for our trip. Thank goodness for my uncle and my ability to match current situations with relevant memories.

Episodic memory also involves future experiences. Whenever something important happens, if you have good episodic memory, you will be storing those memories for future retrieval. You may say to yourself, "This is important! I better remember this." Or if you have ever made a big mistake, you probably learned from it immediately because you didn't want to make the same mistake twice. For example, have you ever started a new job and underestimated your commute time? If you don't like being late, chances are you remembered to leave earlier the next day, because your future episodic memory kicked in and told you to plan differently. Yes, episodic memory will even help you keep your new job.

Episodic memory is vital to social competence. We need it to feel equipped when faced with a problem. We need it to manage a new situation. And we need it to become independent in life.

Episodic memory is vital to social competence. We need it to feel equipped when faced with a problem. We need it to manage a new situation. And we need it to be independent in life.

Here are some examples where we can help kids with social learning challenges strengthen their episodic memory in the moment.

I remember last time you forgot your homework at school we emailed your teacher. In this situation you are helping the student recall that they have experienced this problem in the past, and they have a solution that worked. Your language guides them to retrieve the memory at the moment they need it. As kids gain experience with this type of opportunity, consider fading your language further by saying something like *I remember this has happened before and we figured out a good plan. I'm wondering if you remember too...?* If the child doesn't remember, that is okay. Add more information to help their recall, with the intention of solidifying those memories for the next time around: *Well... I remember we emailed your teacher. Let's try that again.*

In contrast, the imperative might be, *What are you going to do about your homework?* This puts pressure on the child to come up with an answer or solution that may not be at their fingertips, and it might create a perceived threat and activate the fight/flight/freeze response. This is not what we want! Remember to invite and guide the child to recall a similar situation in a positive, supportive way.

This reminds me of a game you already know. For this example, imagine the child does not want to play a new game. They are stuck and not open to the novelty of the situation. What they are not seeing is that, although the game *is* different, many games have similar patterns. It is the predictable pattern of games that make new ones easy enough to learn. In the moment, the child with social learning challenges may focus on the differences, but with your guiding, declarative statements, you can instead emphasize the similarities. This can help the child feel more comfortable trying something new.

To illustrate this idea, think of Candyland and Chutes and Ladders. They are different games, but think of all the ways that they are similar. A piece moves along a path toward a final destination. How many games are like this? Many! Illuminating these similarities can help a child feel less anxious and more ready to join.

In contrast, an imperative approach might be, *Play this game*, or even prompting each of the steps during the game: *Put your piece here, Spin the spinner, Move your piece, Take a card*, etc. If we prompt every step as a child plays the game, without giving them a chance to see that they probably do already know the pattern, we are robbing them of an opportunity to access and use their episodic memory.

Here is one last example.

Have you ever observed kids fight over who is going to go first? Thought so. Instead of trying to stop the arguing, use declarative language to encourage kids to recall shared memories of their play. For example, you could say, *I remember Johnny went first when we played the last game, so I'm thinking it would be most fair to let David go first this time...* You can then also plant seeds for future retrieval; *Let's remember together that when we start another game, it will be Johnny's turn to go first again.*

In contrast, the imperative language in this situation might focus on the challenging behavior (arguing) and trying to stop it (*Stop arguing, No arguing*, etc.). Imperative language would not help the child see the larger pattern at work over the course of time: we all generally do our best to be fair and take turns as we go. The knowledge of this social pattern is what will help them in future peer interactions and play opportunities.

Imperative language would not help the child see the larger pattern at work over the course of time: we all generally do our best to be fair and take turns as we go. The knowledge of this social pattern is what will help them in future peer interactions and play opportunities.

Remember that you can improve social competence by helping kids access and use their episodic memory in the moment. Help them recall what is relevant, while also helping them to store important memories for the future. The next time you notice yourself jumping in to solve a problem for a child or telling them what to do, try to stop yourself. Instead, use declarative comments that invite them to recall a similar but different situation from their past. And from there, guide them to the solution.

CHAPTER 5:
Appreciating Different Opinions

For kids with social learning challenges, taking the perspective of others is a common area of difficulty. As you work to improve an individual's perspective taking abilities, you may feel the need to make them see things your way. But consider again the fight/flight/ freeze response that can be triggered in the face of a perceived threat. If we push too hard, forcing kids to accept or see things that they may not be able to see naturally, we can activate the fight/flight/ freeze response. As a result, kids may become defensive and, instead of being open to our viewpoint, they dig in their heels even more. The result is conflict and negative exchanges as views diverge. This is not what we want. Fortunately, there is a better way!

We don't want to force our views on kids. Instead, we want to create an environment where kids can lower their guard and feel safe to be curious about the thoughts, opinions, and feelings of others. We must create a positive backdrop so that kids do not feel threatened when others have a different thought, opinion, or feeling. We want them to discover, at their own pace, that opinions and perspectives are not right or wrong. They are just different. We want kids to understand that I can think one way while you think another, and this does not mean we are enemies. We can share space and hear what each other has said, respect it, and allow this to strengthen our relationship. As we find our mutual connections, it feels comfortable. But as we discover interesting differences, it helps us grow. We develop friendships and relationships that are interesting because two people are never completely the same.

We must create a positive backdrop so that kids do not feel threatened when others have a different thought, opinion or feeling. We want them to discover, at their own pace, that opinions and perspectives are not right or wrong. They are just different.

So, how do we help kids who may be naturally defensive in this area of different opinions, get to a place of openness? The answer is to truly model being open. Show that you can share space and be with the child through the ups and downs of different opinions, without judgement. Give kids many opportunities to hear your language as you notice different opinions, and as a result, many opportunities to feel safe in that space. Give kids experience disagreeing with you while observing that all is okay. Show how you won't have a big emotional response when they think differently about something. Show how you will note it, and embrace it.

Here are some example statements where you can help kids practice these ideas.

We think differently about that! Imagine you and your child are talking about a certain book or TV show. Maybe you love it and your child is lukewarm. Or it is something that the child loves, but it is just not your thing! Notice this out loud with a simple declarative statement that models interest and respect, and doesn't try to change anyone's mind. By saying, *We think differently about that*, you are also modeling that it is okay to think differently. You show how to stay connected even though you now have an interesting difference between you. You are demonstrating for the child this difference is okay. At the same time, you are also helping the child get to know you better. This is great for building relationships moving forward.

Wow! You are a big Lego fan. We're different that way! Again, you are showing how it is okay to enjoy different things or have different special interests. Just because you are into Legos, Star Wars or whatever, and I am not doesn't mean that we can't have a relationship. As you use these types of comments, you are also incidentally helping kids increase their self-awareness. Too often kids with social learning challenges may not have a clear understanding of what they like, what they don't like, or what makes them unique. Perhaps they have some underlying understanding, or their preferences and comfort levels are revealed through their fight/flight/freeze responses. But wouldn't it be better if they could use language to confidently express who they are? Making declarative statements to kids that describe what we remember about them, will help them learn the language to later use on their own.

I wonder if your buddy likes pretzels as much as you do. This type of statement invites curiosity about another person's opinion in a comfortable, nonthreatening way. This statement does not demand that the child ask if their friend likes pretzels, nor does it communicate judgement on pretzel preferences. Rather, it is a statement that will plant seeds of curiosity in the child's mind about another person. This is what we want.

This type of statement often guides the child to first think: "I don't know," which can then lead them to spontaneously ask their buddy, "Do you like pretzels?" Yes, the declarative statement leads a child to initiate an exchange to learn more about what another person thinks. How cool is that! This is what will take them further in life—genuine curiosity about what other people think. This is what helps them grow, and what can guide kids outside of their comfort zone. It helps to make connections with others and build relationships.

Here are two activities that can foster this idea of opinion sharing, when presented in a declarative way: Essential Oils and Music Clips. With these activities you start with several samples ready and then introduce each (an oil or a music clip) one at a time. Then invite opinions. Wonder together what each person might think about that smell or that sound. Thoughtfully use language that lets kids know it is interesting to hear what other people think or feel, and it is wonderful that these opinions are likely going to be different some of the time.

Because each item may be less familiar, the kids may not yet have the type of fully developed personal opinions that can lead to defensive feelings and strong emotional reactions. Instead, this can be an open, inviting activity where kids can share what they think about a unique smell or sound clip for the first time. As you slow down and move through this activity, leave space for each opinion to be heard and embraced, while also celebrating both the matches and the differences.

I have also found it helpful to structure this activity loosely using what I call an "opinion grid." All you need is a piece of paper and a pencil. Draw a table with columns for each person's name and rows for each oil or song clip. Take your time and write down each person's reaction to the item, pausing to notice whether you have the same or different opinions about each one. (See page 35 for an example).

Here is an example from a girls' group that I lead. The girls in the group were growing their friendships nicely when we realized Elizabeth felt hurt each time her peer, Heidi, had a different opinion

34

on what game to play or activity to do. We introduced this activity to help the girls see that their friendship could handle different opinions, and ultimately be stronger because of it. It definitely helped. However, as the girls grow, we do have to revisit this topic periodically.

OPINION GRID

Write down everyone's reactions or opinions about the scents you smell!

Name → Scent ↓	Linda	Heidi	Elizabeth	Charlotte
Sweet Orange	LOVE it!!	Mmmm nice!	I'm not sure	Yum!
Lavender	Ew. Not for me!	It's okay.	Yuck!	I like it!
Rosemary				

Download a copy of the Opinion Grid at www.declarativelanguage.com

---

Gradually, show kids that we all have similarities which connect us, and differences that help our relationship grow.

Keep in mind that as your child communicates an opinion in some way—be it verbally or through body language—use that moment as an opportunity to show how you can stay connected even when you think differently. Use declarative language to name their feeling or opinion in the moment: *Wow! You are really a fan of XYZ!* Then, make a declarative statement that names your opinion and whether it is the same or different: *I feel totally different about that than you do – how interesting!* Gradually show them that we all have similarities which connect us, and differences that help our relationship grow.

CHAPTER 6:
Making Mistakes is Okay

This is such an important area for kids with social learning challenges. Many kids I know are hard on themselves when it comes to making mistakes. They fear being wrong, and feel awful when they realize they have made a mistake of some sort. This discomfort with mistakes can be crippling. For example, they may not try new things or move outside of their comfort zone, because they don't want to enter a situation where they are unsure what to do, and therefore may make a mistake. As a result, their opportunity for growth and learning becomes significantly limited.

For some kids, a fight/flight/freeze response may be triggered upon realizing that they are wrong in some way. They may have an emotional outburst that takes a while to recover from. They may argue that they are not wrong. They may shut down and turn inward, experiencing increased feelings of sadness about themselves.

How can we help kids feel okay making mistakes? This acceptance is crucial for learning, growing, and feeling comfortable with themselves.

First, if we want to help kids become better at handling their own mistakes – accepting, responding to, and managing them – we, as their teachers in life, must be okay with them *making* mistakes. It is our responsibility to allow mistakes to happen in a safe context, so that kids can develop skill and confidence in fixing mistakes. The use of errorless learning, where a child is prompted to give the right answer within a few seconds, works against this goal. Errorless learning reinforces the idea that it is not acceptable to make mistakes. Can you imagine how stressful it would be if each time you made a mistake someone swooped in to correct you in a matter of seconds? How disheartening. We must give kids time and space to make mistakes, so that they become comfortable with mistakes, and ultimately feel competent fixing them.

It is our responsibility to allow mistakes to happen in a safe context, so that kids can develop skill and confidence in fixing mistakes.

Here are a few examples from some of my favorite perfectionists.

First, my son Desmond! He came home from first grade one day, upset about a paper in his folder. It had the word "great" written ten times in his handwriting. When I asked him about it, he adamantly told me that he did NOT want to talk about it. I gently probed and eventually he shared that he had spelled the word "great" G-R-A-T-E. His teacher proceeded to show him the accurate spelling on their classroom Word Wall, and because it was a commonly misspelled word, she had him write it 10 times to help it stick. Well, his defenses went up fast! He argued with me about how his spelling made more sense—providing solid evidence such as "meat" and "late." I agreed with him! But I explained it's just one of those things, and the word great was on the Word Wall for a reason. It is a tricky word and most kids make mistakes spelling it. Eventually he started to feel better, but that one mistake was painful to him on a deep level.

Chapter 6: Making Mistakes is Okay

I think of another child I know well, Jack. I remember watching Jack and his father, Gary, make Valentine's Day cards for his classmates in third grade. As Jack carefully spelled out each name, his father sat alongside him in a kind, supportive way, letting him carefully form the letters and yes, make mistakes. As he spelled one name, "Madison," Gary noticed he had spelled it with an 'e' instead of an 'i'. Once Jack finished, he looked to his dad to check in, and Gary ever so gently said, "I think Madison has an 'i' instead of an 'e'." Jack's face showed immediate surprise and fear. You could see his thoughts race: what was he going to do about that mistake on the Valentine? Luckily, Gary had been practicing declarative language! He used a declarative statement to remind Jack he was using a pencil and could erase his mistake and fix it. Jack's face relaxed as relief washed over him.

Declarative statements, and the timing of their delivery, are important when it comes to repairing mistakes. If Gary had intervened as soon as he noticed Jack's mistake, the flow of Jack's work would have been interrupted. Jack would've been corrected in the middle of the task, which would likely have decreased his confidence in moving forward. Instead, Gary waited until Jack had finished the name, and waited for the moment when Jack naturally checked in for guidance. Gary knew that Jack would be ready at that point to handle the new information (there was a correction to be made) and subsequently would also be ready to take on problem solving with renewed energy.

In that moment, Gary did something more important than teaching Jack how to spell Madison. He showed Jack that it was perfectly fine to make a mistake, because he knew Jack had the tools to fix it. This life lesson can be applied across numerous contexts and will build Jack's confidence moving forward. This is what was most important.

Since that day, Jack has in fact gone on to move outside his comfort zone in many ways. I'm sure the guiding style of his parents, which allowed him to make mistakes, helped this growth happen. For example, Jack ran for student council in middle school and won! Prior to voting day, he had to stand in front of his middle school classmates and give a speech. Being able to do this illustrates his personal growth into someone who does not let the fear of mistakes control his choices.

These are the skills we want to develop. Not reckless abandon, but we want our kids with social learning challenges to bravely move outside their comfort zone. We want them to feel comfortable trying new things, and to spontaneously seek out new challenges and growth opportunities. To do this, they must be ready to handle learning in all its forms, which includes mistakes. The more kids experience mistakes and feel their own ability to handle those mistakes improving, their resilience grows. You'll see this change happen as they become less upset, more open, and recover more quickly when making a mistake.

So now let's tie this teaching to declarative language. Start to really notice the small mistakes that you make every day. Demystify mistakes by commenting on them in the presence of your child, while also talking about how you felt at the time, how you handled the situation, and how you fixed things.

Here are some everyday examples.

You took a wrong turn while driving. Say this out loud so your child can hear what happened: *Oops! I took a wrong turn. I need to turn the car around. It's okay, we will still get to where we need to be.*

Or when in the kitchen:
Oh man! I just spilled the milk. That's okay. I'll grab a paper towel.

Oh, I'm sorry! I thought you said you did want blueberries on your cereal. My bad!

It is powerful when we can model an observation of our own mistake and then model how we take responsibility for it. I try to say, "My bad!" often when I'm around kids, including my own. I want them to see and hear that no one is perfect, and we are all learning to manage our own mistakes.

It is powerful when we can model an observation of our own mistake and then model how we take responsibility for it.

I mentioned this previously in the example with Jack, but it is important enough to mention again. When you are guiding kids to notice and manage their own mistakes, it is important to slow your pace. You should allow the child the opportunity to realize the mistake on their own. Discovery is an essential part of the process. It is much easier to fix and feel comfortable with a mistake when you discover it on your own. And it is reassuring when someone you know and trust is there to help if needed.

So when you see your child make a mistake, try to wait quietly. Let them discover it first, and then let them know you are there to help if needed. If your child does not notice the mistake, then guide their observation through a declarative statement. Some examples:

I think that word has an 'e' in it.
It might be a good idea to check number 2 again.
Oh! I see some of that water spilled.
Hmmm... Let's take another look at where you placed that Lego.

When you see your child make a mistake, try to wait quietly. Let them discover it first, and then let them know you are there to help if needed.

Next, don't butt in and correct the mistake. Simply use a declarative statement to guide the discovery of the mistake and wait. Once the child notices it, give them space to fix it on their own. Let them work it out for a few moments. This is where active problem-solving skills develop.

For example, let them notice the spilled water, and then pause. I bet they might come up with an idea to clean it up on their own. Or if you guide them to re-check math problem #2, chances are they will find their mistake and then fix it on their own.

However, if the problem is bigger than the child's current toolbox and you wait, they will likely then visually reference you for guidance, because you have quietly waited for them to invite you. You have helped preserve their personal agency, and now that they are ready for help, you can successfully expand their toolbox around that opportunity.

In groups at our clinic, we focus a lot on the idea of "Making Mistakes is Okay." In fact, on some vacation weeks we dedicate a special two-day camp to that idea alone. We used declarative statements to teach kids how some mistakes turned into important discoveries (potato chips, chocolate chip cookies, etc.), that mistakes can be funny ("Did I tell you about the time my sister wore two different shoes to school by mistake?"), how we can sometimes create something new out of mistakes, and how mistakes, although embarrassing at times, inevitably help us learn and grow. There are many books out there on this topic, as well, that are fun and interesting to read with kids. *Amelia Bedelia* by Peggy Parish, *Beautiful Oops* by Barney Saltzberg, *Mistakes that Worked* by Charlotte Foltz Jones, *Don't be Afraid to Drop!* by Julia Cook, *Your Fantastic, Elastic Brain: Stretch It, Shape It* by JoAnn Deak and *The Most Magnificent Thing* by Ashley Spires are a few titles that I read often.

As we end this chapter, keep in mind these declarative statements that empower kids around mistakes:

I am sure you can handle that mistake!
That mistake made me laugh.
Let's see how we can fix this. I bet we can do it together.
I remember making this mistake before. I can help if you need it.
I bet you will figure this out. I am here if you need me.

Remember, the next time you observe your child make a mistake, or they are about to make a mistake, don't jump in quickly to correct them. If it is not a safety issue, allow them time to make the mistake so they can learn how to fix it. This will help them become comfortable with the feelings associated with making mistakes. If we correct too quickly or never let kids make mistakes, how do we expect them to manage mistakes in the real world? Use your declarative statements in the moment to be emotionally supportive, patient, and guiding when teaching kids how to navigate mistakes.

CHAPTER 7:
Thinking in Alternatives and Possibilities

The next important area to help kids with social learning challenges is related to problem solving—thinking in terms of alternatives and possibilities. Many concrete or black and white thinkers are comfortable solving problems in one specific way. As you can imagine, it can become stressful when their "go-to" way of doing things is not possible or doesn't work out. They may become worried and insist on doing things the usual way. This worry may be communicated through a challenging behavior – arguing, not moving, a tantrum, etc. When faced with this situation, a teacher or caregiver's first instinct may be to force a change in behavior. Behavior change is fine, but where we can make the biggest impact in the long term is to address the problem at the point of thinking. If we can help kids think more flexibly about the problem, then that will lead to more flexible responses. We want kids with social learning challenges to think positively about the possibilities of any situation, rather than get stuck because they feel they have hit a dead end.

Here's an example to illustrate thinking in alternatives or possibilities.

Imagine you come outside to go to work in the morning and you have a flat tire. First, you don't freak out because you have good episodic memory and can think of many solutions in the moment. You brainstorm: Should I call AAA? Should I walk? Should I take a taxi? A bus? Call a friend? You think through all the possible solutions you have either experienced on your own or that you have knowledge of in response to a flat tire. After brainstorming possible solutions, you pick the best one. This is what alternative thinking is: thinking of many possible ideas and deciding which is the best fit for right now. This is what we want to help our kids get better at.

In order to work on this skill with kids, recognize that it is best not to target it in the moment of stress. Rather, it is much better to model possibilities of how this type of thinking works when the stakes are low. Your first goal is simply to help kids be open to thinking about many ideas versus only one. They don't need to decide yet. They only need to hear what you are thinking.

Here are some examples of how to use declarative language to get this thinking going.

You are walking to the playground and think aloud using this declarative statement: *Maybe we could walk a different way than we usually do today...*

Or you are driving to school and comment, *Oh! Road work. Looks like we need to take a detour.*

In school, imagine kids working on a project related to the ocean. They each need to use a big piece of blue paper. But you notice a problem and share it using a declarative statement: *Oops! There is only one piece of blue paper left. How about if kids use white paper with blue paint, or green paper instead.*

After you have started modeling alternative thinking, engage kids in brainstorming when possible. This requires slowing down to invite ideas. When brainstorming, I like to tell kids, "Every idea is good enough to write down." I say this because some kids hesitate to write down an idea when they feel it is not perfect. They worry it is not good enough and don't want to commit while still searching for something better. But here's what's important: writing down all ideas, even the ones that may be considered subpar, gets everyone's creative juices flowing. When you tell them that all of their ideas are good enough to write down, if you notice kids are hesitating, be sure to add this declarative statement: *You don't have to use what you've written unless you want to.* Tell them that the act of brainstorming itself begets more ideas. Help them get to a place where they feel brave enough to brainstorm and experience the joy that follows when ideas flow.

When brainstorming, I like to tell kids, "Every idea is good enough to write down." Help them get to a place where they feel brave enough to brainstorm so they can experience the joy that follows when ideas flow.

When brainstorming, it is always equally important for caregivers and teachers to make declarative statements that communicate an openness to all ideas contributed. Even if they seem out of the ordinary at first. For example, you can always say, *Wow! What an interesting idea!* Embrace and respect ideas so kids feel safe enough to keep going.

When brainstorming, it is always equally important for caregivers and teachers to make declarative statements that communicate an openness to all ideas contributed. Even if they seem out of the ordinary at first.

Remember my earlier example of Eliza and her wooden dolls? I started the brainstorming process with a comment: *I wonder what that could be...* while we explored a piece of material around the doll's neck. In my mind it was a necktie. But I stayed silent after my declarative statement and was so glad I did. Eliza had an idea that was different from mine and fantastic. In that moment I saw the power of declarative language because it invites ideas from everyone, and we all benefit from the alternatives we weren't expecting.

When getting started at home, use incidental moments throughout the day to practice alternative thinking. There are likely many moments when you typically plow ahead and make decisions without a word to your child. But if you slow down, pause, and invite ideas using declarative language, you are teaching important social learning lessons in a positive way. You are making a process that is usually elusive, transparent to our black and white thinkers. For example, you could say *Hmmm... I'm trying to decide whether we should walk or bike to the library today* or *We need to take the recycling bins out to the curb. I wonder if we should do it tonight or tomorrow morning.*

You can also show that alternative ideas can be fun! For example, invite everyone to consider sitting in different seats at the dinner table because... why not? *Let's all try a different seat tonight!* Or consider what having dessert before dinner might be like: *I wonder what it would be like to have dessert first!* What if you eat breakfast foods for dinner? *Hey! I have a funny idea for dinner tonight!* There are many playful ways to change things up to illustrate the benefits of embracing possibility. If any of these possibilities cause stress in your child, don't force it. Simply model the idea yourself by saying something like *I know you don't want to do this right now. That's okay! But I'm going to give it a try.*

Here are some additional declarative comments that target thinking in alternatives and possibilities:

Hmmm…I wonder what topping we could add to our pancakes this morning!

I notice we are out of staples. I'm wondering what we could use instead.

Oh no! The door is locked. I'm wondering how we could get inside if our usual way is not working. I wonder what we could do instead.

Remember, the easier it becomes to think of new or different ideas, the more relaxed a person will feel because their eggs are not all in one basket. When thinking in terms of possibility, it is always easy to find a solution when things don't go as planned. In contrast, when a child only has one idea or one plan, fight/flight/freeze responses kick in when that one way doesn't work or is not possible. They feel stress, get upset, and their problem-solving brain goes out the window. Use declarative statements to get alternative thinking started, invite idea sharing, and embrace contributions.

PART 3

MECHANICS

The Nuts and Bolts—Constructing Declarative Statements

We have been talking a lot about the various social learning benefits that can be gained as you become comfortable using declarative language. Now let's review the definition of declarative language itself and get down to the nuts and bolts of constructing these types of statements so you become a pro!

As a review, imperative language places demands on kids to do or say something. In contrast, declarative language *invites* them. Imperative language consists of commands and questions with a right or wrong answer. Declarative language is a series of statements or comments with no correct or incorrect response.

Sometimes when people get started, they ask kids a lot of questions, thinking this is declarative language. It is not. Please always keep in mind that questions are not declarative language. The question may contain a great idea, but for it to be declarative, you must shape it into a comment. Questions place additional processing and formulation demands on kids, making it harder for them to respond.

Declarative statements smoothly guide them. Get in the habit of changing questions into comments.

Questions are not declarative language. The question may contain a great idea, but for it to be declarative, you must shape it into a comment.

Here are some example questions that I hear a lot:

What should you do?
What are you missing?
What do you need?

These are all great beginning ideas because you are inviting the child to notice something and act. But because they are questions, there are too many demands. Let's change them into comments:

What should you do? → *I'm wondering what you should do* or *I think now is a good time to do X.*
What are you missing? → *I notice you are missing something* or *I think you need your shoes!*
What do you need? → *It's time for math. You need a few things!* Or *It's time for math. You'll need your pencil and your book.*

Next, when constructing declarative statements, here are some tips. Declarative language has great variety, so don't feel like you must use all the ideas at once! Depending on what you want to say, use these ideas as a guide for how to say it best.

1. **Make simple comments that observe and invite the child to observe too.**

These comments will guide the child to integrate information from their environment. Examples:

- *The dog looks hungry!* Here you are inviting the child to notice the dog, notice an empty bowl, put those things together and realize, "Aha! I need to feed the dog." Then the child can problem solve around how to go about it. This is very different than the imperative: "Feed the dog" or even the question that places demands, "What does the dog need?"

- *Those flowers are pretty.* Imagine you are on a walk with your child. By commenting on observations that you share while you walk, you are helping them to remember something interesting about your walk and creating a shared memory that you can talk about later. You are also modeling communication for joint attention, which kids with social learning challenges may not naturally use on their own. This is important because if we want kids to get better at sharing their experiences (which creates social connections), we have to show them how to do it!

2. **Use cognitive verbs, or verbs that model our thinking.**

These verbs help kids reach higher levels of discourse, problem solving, and social connection. With these verbs, you are helping kids go beyond the concrete and showing them there is a thought process behind all we do. Kids who struggle with flexible thinking or perspective taking don't know this intuitively. Our thoughtful language modeling in this regard will show them how it's done, and help them better understand the actions and intentions of others. We will show them how people usually *think* before *acting*. Examples of cognitive verbs include:

Declarative Language Handbook

- Think
- Wonder
- Remember
- Forget
- Know
- Imagine
- Decide
- Wish

Quick tip: Anytime you hear yourself ask a question, you can easily turn it into a declarative by taking out the question word (e.g., what, why, where, etc.) and replacing it with "I wonder."

Example: *What do you need to do?* can become *I wonder if you know what to do.*

Here is one of my favorite stories to illustrate how these thinking verbs, when embedded in declarative statements, get to a higher level of discourse. A 9-year-old boy named Michael hated when it rained. He loved to go outside for recess and when it rained, he couldn't. In fact, whenever it was rainy, he would arrive at school saying, "It's not raining!" His teachers tried to get him to say otherwise, and when he wouldn't, they concluded he was being rigid.

One day it dawned on me that Michael was likely having trouble expressing what he meant. I knew he knew it was raining. That was not the issue. So I said, "Michael, I wonder if you mean you *wish* it wasn't raining." Immediately he answered, "Yes! I wish it wasn't raining." And with that simple addition to his statement, we could move beyond the misinterpretation that he was being rigid, and towards fostering greater social connection and teaching the nuances of language. This was an opportunity to learn more about Michael's thoughts, opinions, and feelings, and help him expand his vocabulary so that he could better express these to others. It was also an opportunity to help him problem solve.

After he acknowledged what he really meant, I then said to him, "I know Michael. It's hard when it rains out. Most kids don't like it. Most kids feel that way because they can't go outside and have to think of different things to do during recess time." Immediately, our conversation touched on the experience he was having and validated his feelings. It then moved on to problem solving: "Michael, let's think of some things that you could do at recess when it rains. It won't be the same as going outside, but maybe it will be good enough."

The declarative statement created a space for Michael to express his feelings and then guided him toward problem solving. This conversation was richer, more dynamic, and more meaningful than the previous debate about what the sky was doing.

The declarative statement created a space for Michael to express his feelings and then guided him toward problem solving. The conversation became richer, more dynamic and more meaningful.

---

3. **Use words that emphasize uncertainty and possibility.**

Remember in the previous chapter how I talked about helping kids to think in terms of alternative and possibility? These words help make it happen. As you begin to use these types of words naturally in conversation, you will create opportunities for the child to become comfortable with uncertainty, gray areas, and the idea of not knowing something. Here are some of those types of words and phrases:

- Maybe
- Might
- Possibly
- Perhaps
- Sometimes
- I'm sure/not sure
- I don't know

Examples of declarative statements with these words:
We might go to the store later.
Maybe we should check the weather.
It might be rainy tomorrow.
Perhaps there is another way to do this.
Sometimes it can help to use a pencil instead of a pen.
As you make these statements, feel how you are moving away from one specific idea and moving towards possibility.

4. **Use words that communicate your own uncertainty and that acknowledge what you don't know.**

Making thoughts about your own uncertainty transparent will help kids who fear being wrong. Your willingness to "not know" something shows kids that this is normal. When I don't know something, I seize the opportunity to say to kids, *That's a great question. I don't know the answer yet.* Or *I'm not sure about that. What a great thought!* I want kids to also get comfortable in this space. They may not be able to admit not knowing something at first, but with thoughtful modeling, you can create a place for them where it is safe to not know something.

Your willingness to "not know" something shows kids that this is normal.

---

5. **Use words related to your feelings or senses, and words that help kids observe their environment.**

We observe with our eyes, but we also observe with our other senses. Imagine what you are guiding the child to observe by using these declarative statements:

I notice it is getting cloudy.
I see that the teacher is ready for us to start.
Your mom looks upset!
I think I smell pizza!
There is a smell coming from the cafeteria right now. I wonder what's for lunch.
I heard something.
I heard the doorbell.
I can hear him laughing. I think he is happy about that!
I heard your friend say something.

This last example is important because it invites kids to notice a communication breakdown (their friend said something, and they missed it) and leaves space for them to repair it. Repairing a communication breakdown is a vital communication skill. It is problems solving in action. In response to your comment, the child might think, "Oh! He did? Let me find out what he said," thereby taking ownership. In contrast, an imperative such as, *What did your friend say?* or *Ask your friend what he said* does not give the child the same opportunity to observe what has happened. When you help kids notice

55

communication breakdowns by pointing out what they have missed, without fixing the problem for them, you help them develop important communication skills. If they need help or further guidance, it is always okay to provide this (more on that in Chapter 10 and Chapter 11), but as a first response, comment and then wait quietly for the child to notice, think, and act on their own.

When you help kids notice communication breakdowns by pointing out what they have missed, without fixing the problem for them, you help them develop vital communication skills.

---

6. **Use inviting first person pronouns to help kids engage and join you.**
   Instead of telling kids what to do, emphasize a partnership using first person plural pronouns such as *let's, we,* and *us.*

Examples:

Let's get ready to go out.
We could go to the movies.
This project will be interesting for us to do!

By using first-person singular pronouns such as *I, my, mine,* and *me,* you can thoughtfully model an idea or opinion without putting pressure on the child. You are thinking through an idea and showing them what to do, but because you are the one doing it, you are creating a place for the child to observe and then decide on their own what to do. Examples:

Chapter 8: The Nuts and Bolts

I'm going to put on my shoes now.
My idea is to play Scrabble.
I can't wait to see Grandpa.
Here is my pencil. I'm going to use it to write my name.

As you get comfortable constructing declarative statements, keep in mind that practice helps. Try out the above suggestions at your own pace. If it feels overwhelming, or seems like a lot to remember, it may help to try out each idea on its own for a week. Or you could pick one daily routine with your child such as bedtime, and then slow down and concentrate on your language without worry. As you gain skill and confidence in this new speaking style, you will start to hear yourself seamlessly integrate the ideas. With practice, it will become automatic!

CHAPTER 9:

Is It Ever Okay to Be Imperative?

We have been talking so much about the benefits of declarative language that it sometimes can be overwhelming to figure out where and when to get started. Especially if this is a big shift for you! What I want you to know is that learning to speak in a declarative way is a process. It doesn't happen overnight, and it can be hard work to change your speaking style. But it is possible, and it is worth it. It becomes easier and more automatic the more you do it. I promise!

As people get excited about the change, I am often asked if or when it would be okay to use imperative language. I will answer this question but first I want to share what I have noticed. People become the most imperative when they feel in a hurry. For example, getting kids ready and out the door in the morning can be a very imperative time. Even in my house. We feel the time pressure and must get those kids moving! Busy times do not always allow us to slow down in the way we need to for declarative language to be successful.

So, as you take your first steps with declarative language, don't try to do it at times when you know you will feel stressed and rushed. Instead, pick a time in your week or day where you can let go, pause, and allow yourself to make statements, without pressure. It is your time to practice. You carve it out, plan for it, and do it. You don't even need to tell anyone. During these practice times, I bet you will notice changes in the overall communication patterns between you and your child. You will be able to breathe, and you will notice their unique responses. Enjoy it!

Having said that, here are three times when it's alright to consider imperative language.

With regards to safety – We can't let our kids get into situations that are not safe. If there is a safety issue and time is of the essence, you may need to use an imperative to get the message quickly to the child. For example, *Get down, Hold my hand,* or *Don't run* might be necessary imperatives at certain times.

When setting limits – Contrary to what you may think, you don't need to be imperative to set limits or be firm with kids. There are declarative statements that do this too. But the difference between an imperative and declarative when setting limits, is that the declarative provides the child with important social information and your perspective, as well as the limit you need to set. Imperatives only tell kids what to do (or not do). It is up to you in the moment to decide how much information the child can realistically hear, process, and respond to. Sometimes you may start with a declarative and then realize the child needs more direct language in that moment. Here are some examples to show the contrast:

- Declarative: *It is important that you hold my hand in the parking lot.*
- Imperative: *Hold my hand.*

- Declarative: *I don't want you to run right now because it is not safe.*
- Imperative: *Don't run.*

- Declarative: *I will feel upset if you keep doing that.*
- Imperative: *Please stop!*

As I mentioned, you can be firm using a declarative statement. The benefit to using the declarative is that you are giving the child more information, which will help them understand the context. Often when we give kids that extra information, they acquiesce because they now understand the reasoning behind the limit.

The benefit to using the declarative when setting a limit is that you are giving the child more information, which will help them understand the context. Often when we give kids that extra information, they acquiesce because they now understand the reasoning behind the limit.

While you are learning – It is of course okay to be imperative while you learn to speak declaratively! Don't be too hard on yourself. The most important thing in this process is that you are starting to think about your speaking style and beginning to understand how powerful saying things in a different way can be. Also know that you can make mistakes.

As you hear yourself use an imperative where a declarative would've been possible, take that moment to rephrase what you have said. It is great for your own learning to make that repair in the moment. For example, if you hear yourself say, *What did I say?* take a moment to pause and rephrase: *I'm sorry. I meant to say, I'm wondering if you heard what I said?* Or if you hear yourself say, *Turn off the TV* or *Come to the table*, pause and rephrase: *I'd love it if you would turn off the TV now because it's time for dinner.*

Start small and be mindful. That is what it is all about. Your mindfulness in speaking will carry over and show your kids the power of communication, and that they can be thoughtful too. Try to move away from having imperative language be your first response. You can use imperatives if you need to, but start to notice all the times that you don't! If a declarative statement doesn't seem to work, then you can try out some troubleshooting tips, which I will discuss in Chapter 11.

Most importantly, however, when people ask me about imperative language, this is what I say:

Many people speak to kids with social learning challenges using imperative language because they think they need it. They may need it sometimes, but there are many times that they probably don't. In fact, imperative language is not the speaking style that will teach them what they most need to learn.

Kids with social learning challenges need and can benefit from the richness of declarative language. So, your goal is not to pick one style of speaking over the other. Your goal is to be thoughtful and use imperative language when you need it, but don't use it when you don't.

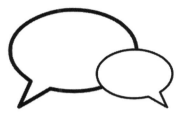

PART 4:

PACING AND TROUBLESHOOTING

The Importance of Pacing

A most important partner to declarative language use is pacing. "Pacing" means slowing down your delivery of information enough for the child to effectively process what you have said and respond. Starting out, this means you deliver one unit of information and then wait. You are waiting so you can observe the child's cues. You are waiting for them to indicate that they have received the message. Their cues may be verbal or nonverbal.

"Pacing" means slowing down your delivery of information enough for the child to effectively process what you have said and respond.

Some cues that you may see include a visual reference, as discussed in Chapter 3. The child may look to you if they need further guidance or if they feel unsure. Or they may look to the surrounding environment to see what you have just commented upon. Another cue is them acting upon what you have said. For example, if you said, *Your shirt is on the floor* and the child responds by putting it in the hamper, that is the cue that your message was received!

The important piece here is that you are stating your thought, idea, observation, memory, etc. and then *waiting* for the child to show that they heard and understood. If you jump in too quickly with more information or repeat yourself prematurely, then the child has even more information to process and respond to, and you have been counterproductive. It is worth it to wait!

Another great sign is when you see a child have an "aha" moment, or a discovery. This means that they have processed what you said and have made a realization as a result. These discoveries are empowering and feel good to all. Example: *You dropped something!* (Aha! There it is) and the child picks the item off the floor. These moments are fun to observe.

When I first started using declarative language, I knew waiting was important. I made myself count to at least 30 in my head before saying anything else. I was amazed to observe the power of waiting for the first time and remember it clearly. I was working with three-year-old Eliza. She was coloring and I wanted to color too. Normally I would have said, *Can you get me a marker?* but instead I said, *I would like to color too.* Then I waited and didn't say anything. I counted in my head with the intention of staying quiet until I got to 30. But at around 10 seconds, Eliza got up from her spot next to me on the floor and said, "I can get you a marker." She ran in the other room, got a marker, and brought it back for me to use. I was floored! I didn't know she could infer like that or that she could execute a plan independently, especially one based on something related to my perspective and wishes. And I would never have known had I continued to speak imperatively to her. Pacing and declarative language are important partners. You must try it out!

Chapter 10: The Importance of Pacing

Here is a way to think about pacing and its importance. When we pause, we are allowing the child to integrate all the pieces of information out there. We are providing them space to process what we have said, to notice the environment, to recognize our feelings or their own feelings, to recall relevant memories, and to ultimately make a decision by using all of these factors. It is a complex process, so no wonder time is needed to do it.

Don't ever underestimate the power of waiting quietly. Remember that silence is your friend. You do not need to fill the space—even when it feels awkward. If you need help feeling comfortable in the quiet, remember that you are giving the child time to think. Then put that time to practical use and observe the child. Wait quietly and watch for feedback. Did they hear you? Did they understand what you said? Might they be confused? It is in those moments of silence that you can determine how the message was received and make your own decision around next steps. For example, do they need more help or guidance? Do you need to get closer and repeat what you said? These are some tips that will be expanded upon in the next chapter. If troubleshooting is necessary, you are going to be in the best place for it when you have waited quietly and observed. Quietly receiving feedback helps you to know how to best help the child moving forward.

Don't ever underestimate the power of waiting quietly.

As I mentioned in previous chapters, start slowly with your use of declarative language and choose times and situations when you can be successful. Now that you know how important pacing is, start to practice pacing and declarative language. Pick a scenario when you can allow yourself to slow down enough to count to 30 in your head before you say the next thing. This takes strength for sure, and I want you to gain confidence in your ability to stay quiet when this is called for. Help yourself by choosing a time that you know you won't feel stressed. Choose a time when you can give yourself permission to slow down, breath, and say one thing at a time, while observing your child's cues.

Here are some examples to illustrate the balance of statements and pauses.

Example 1:

I wonder what you have for homework tonight. Pause for processing time. After 10 seconds Matthew has his "aha" moment. He gets his backpack and opens it to look in his planner.

I wonder what you have for homework tonight. Pause for processing time. After 10 seconds Matthew looks up and says to you, "I don't know." You then add another declarative statement because he has provided you feedback and is ready for more information: *It might be a good idea to get your planner, and we can look at it together.* Pause for processing time. Matthew has his "aha" moment and gets his planner.

I wonder what you have for homework tonight. Pause for processing time. You have counted to 30 in your head and Matthew has not moved. Use a troubleshooting tip from the next chapter.

Example 2:

It is time for work in the Kindergarten classroom, but Clara is still playing in the house corner. You say, *I see that all the kids are at the table, ready for work* and allow for processing time. Clara stops what she is doing, looks over to her table and sees her classmates seated. She has an "aha" moment and goes to the table too.

I see all the kids are at the table, ready for work. Allow for processing time. Clara looks to you and asks, "Can I still play?" You respond with additional declarative comments that validate her feelings, make a plan, and set a limit: *I can see that you love playing with those toys! I bet we can find time to play later, but right now I need you to come to the table.*

I see all the kids are at the table, ready for work Allow for processing time. You have counted to 30 in your head but Clara does not turn around and keeps playing. Use a troubleshooting tip from the next chapter.

In a nutshell, here are possible ways a child will provide feedback:
- They reference their surroundings and take action.
- They reference you, and communicate uncertainty and/or communicate (verbally or nonverbally) a need for further guidance or clarification.
- They do not respond.

Remember, pace the information you share so that the child has time to hear, process, think, and respond. Silence is an important and necessary component of this process. Embrace it and get comfortable becoming an observer. Comment, wait and observe, and provide more information as needed. It's a dance which cannot be predetermined. You must use your observations as your guide.

Also remember to practice during times when you can slow down and hone these important skills. The learning process will remain open and positive as you give kids time to think. Many kids are initially not used to receiving this time to process information. They are used to being rushed or being told what to do! So starting out, they may need more processing time to get used to the new pattern. But as they acclimate to it, and as you do too, things will speed up. The skills of hearing, integrating contextual information, and acting on it become more comfortable and automatic. Try your best to hold back from saying more or speaking too soon. That will make everything harder because the child will have to restart processing information over again. Embrace your new mantra: Speak, wait quietly, and add more as needed. You can do this!

Practice during times when you can slow down and hone these important skills. The learning process will remain open and positive as you give kids time to think.

CHAPTER 11:
Troubleshooting Tips

Now that you are excited to give declarative language a try (or have already started!), you have more than likely run into some trouble spots. For example, maybe you have made a few comments here and there and your child has not responded. You may be thinking, "Hey this doesn't work!" But wait and be assured that it is normal and expected for declarative language to not work immediately and/or every time. This is because it is a change, and change takes time. Everyone needs to get used to the new normal.

For you, the change involves your speaking style. But for your child, the change is getting used to the fact that you are not going to prompt them. Their brain may be waiting for the prompt and may need a little time to adjust to the leaps you are asking it to make. They also have to get used to the idea that they now have a bigger responsibility than they did before.

There are common reasons why a child may not respond to your carefully constructed declarative statements. I consider these often and will share the usual suspects in my opinion. I'll start by listing them, but then will explain each in detail along with next steps you can take. As discussed in the previous chapter, you will have to be a thoughtful observer of the individual child to determine which reason makes the most sense in each moment.

- **Processing time** – you jumped in too quickly!
- **Attention** – your child is not attending to your language, for a variety of possible reasons.
- **Comprehension** – your child hears you but does not understand what is expected.
- **Habit** – the child is not used to this speaking style and needs time to adjust.

Let's go through each one.

Processing time – Did you make a declarative comment and then only give a second or two before you prompted again? Remember, this language is different. The child needs to process it, think about it, and then decide how to respond. It is a bit of brain work to do, and adequate processing time is important. If you speak again too quickly, you add more demands and create more work. The child may get overloaded, get stuck, or not know what to do. I know I discussed pacing in the previous chapter so bear with me! I'm mentioning it again here because it remains so very important.

Attention – The message was not received because you didn't have the child's attention. It's not that they don't want to pay attention to you, it's that they were attending to something else when you spoke. It's not that the child is willful. It's not that they don't want to hear you. Trust me. They need you to try again but this time, ensure you have their attention before you speak.

Here are a few ways to secure their attention before making your declarative statement:

1. <u>Get closer to the child and try again.</u> It may just be that the child is too far away, and your voice didn't travel the distance in a way that helps the child know the message is important.

2. <u>Call their name or tap their shoulder.</u> Once you call their name or tap their shoulder you have an important job. I want you to WAIT. Wait until the child has processed this first initial bid. You will know they have successfully processed this initial communication when they reference you. They will either visually reference you (look towards you) or they may verbally reference you by saying "What?" Either way, their reference to you indicates that they are now ready for more information. You want to wait for this signal of readiness, because what you are going to say is important.

3. <u>Hold their attention once you've got it.</u> I also sometimes do double duty in terms of getting and keeping a child's attention by letting them know I have something important to tell them. First, I call their name, wait for them to reference me, and then I add a comment that signals something important is to come. For example, I may say, *I have something important to tell you. Let me know when you are ready,* Or *I want to tell you something. I'll wait until you're ready.* Or even, *I have something exciting to tell you! Let me know when you are ready to hear it.* These statements set you up for success. The child will pause what they are doing, reference you, and then let you know they are ready to take in what you have to say. They are eager to hear you and they are ready. This will increase the likelihood that they will process and respond to your declarative comment. Set yourself up for success by getting their attention in a meaningful way first!

4. <u>Minimize distractions.</u> It also can be helpful to ensure you are not competing with other items in the environment. If the child is not referencing you after you have moved through these above steps to secure their attention, perhaps that Lego they are using or that item that they are holding or thinking

about is too big a competitor for their attention, and you are losing! In this situation, it is best to remove it before you make your comment. You could say, *I can tell you like that toy. I'm going to hold it for a minute while I tell you something important.* Then put your hand out for them to give you the item. Once removed, they are more likely to attend to what you say. Then when they ask for the item back, if some follow-through is needed, you could say, *I will definitely give this back to you, but first I want you to take care of what I just mentioned.* If you only wanted to tell them something, share a memory or give a preview for something coming up, then you should give the item back right way to show that you are trustworthy, and you honor your word.

5. <u>Scan and simplify the environment.</u> Similarly, you want to look for potential distractions in the environment. Get the most bang for your buck by removing potentially distracting items as best you can, before you speak.

6. <u>Make a repair.</u> If you have reduced distractions and feel confident that your child should have heard you, but they haven't responded, use a declarative statement to initiate a communicate repair. For example, using a positive tone of voice, say, *I want to make sure you heard me,* Or *I'm not sure you heard me.* Wait for the child to process what you have said. If your statement was positive and inviting, they will likely respond by self-advocating: "No, I didn't. Can you say it again?"

Comprehension – The third reason a child might not respond to a declarative statement is that they don't know what to do. Perhaps you are presenting a new idea, using less familiar vocabulary, or the child hasn't yet experienced the situation or problem you are presenting.

Perhaps the job or expectation is too big in relation to their current skill set for handling it.

Here is an example that I will walk you through.

Nick was at the grocery store with his mother, Sue. He put milk in the carriage and his mom said, *I wonder if one milk is enough for both you and Daddy.* Nick looked to his mom but did not respond in any way. He was stuck. His visual reference cue indicated he received the message, but it was clear that he did not understand what Sue meant or did not know what she expected him to do next.

When the child does not know what to do, you will have to break down what you are saying into smaller chunks that are understandable to the child, and guide them, one idea at a time.

Any slowing down that you do to break down ideas in this way is time well spent. The learning you provide in these moments will plant seeds for another day. You are helping the child learn something new and store this knowledge for the future. Because you have slowed down to teach, the child will more easily recall what to do when they hear a similar declarative comment again. You are actively working on episodic memory.

When you have slowed down to teach, the child will more easily recall what to do when they hear a similar comment again. You are actively working on episodic memory.

Nick's mother broke down her initial comment and guided Nick with more information so that he could understand and learn: *Maybe you should get one for you and one for Daddy.* Immediately, Nick responded by following through with the suggested actions and grabbing another milk for their cart. You can also be reasonably sure that the next time he hears someone say, *I wonder if that is enough,*

Nick will infer that he should add more. But Sue needed to slow down in that moment to teach the idea.

As you can see, when a child is stuck as to what to do next, it is often that the child simply needs more guiding, more information, more breaking down of the task. Take the time to do this using guiding statements and it will be worth it.

Sometimes parents or teachers backtrack and think they need to ask more questions, *What should you be doing? What do you need?* but be strong and don't ask those questions! Questions will create greater demands. Stay strong and use guiding comments to navigate the child through this less familiar event, and know you are helping them store important memories.

Another way to support comprehension is to add a gesture.

For example, if you say, *I see trash on the floor* and the child hears you but doesn't respond, they may need help locating the trash. Pause, and then add a gesture. For example, point toward the trash, which will successfully guide their attention toward what you want them to see. Or another possibility is that maybe they see the trash on the floor but don't see the trash can. Further guide them using both a point and a comment: *The trash can is right over there.*

Here's another example where a Kindergarten teacher recently asked for my help.

One of her students frequently hid under the table when it was time to do work. The teacher made the declarative statement, *All the kids are sitting in their chairs,* to encourage the student to reference the room and know what was expected. But the student did not budge.

In this moment, the student is likely feeling unsure or worried about expectations. She may be able to sit in the chair, but she may feel unsure if she will be able to do what is expected once she is there!

In this situation, more information about what's to come would be helpful, along with how the child will receive support, if necessary. In this situation, you want to move your focus away from the "get" (How do I get her out from under there?) and move towards a "give" that will help ease her worry. (What information can I give her in this moment that will help?)

The teacher could start by saying, *You can sit right here in your chair. I will help you if you need it.* If the student still doesn't move, she could add, *We are going to be coloring. I see crayons on the table.* If the student is still feeling worried, the teacher could validate her feelings by saying, *I think you may feel nervous about what we're doing, but I will be right here to help. I don't want you to feel worried.*

This inviting language will help the child feel supported and safe, decrease worry, and be more ready to join. Sometimes your first goal may be simply helping the child to join. That is an okay place to start because once they have joined, you can guide further with declarative language.

These examples of guiding statements are all very different from the usual commands and questions that may be used in this type of situation and could create power struggles such as: *What do you need to do? Sit in the chair,* or *Get out from under the table.* With these declarative statements you are creating a very different environment of support, guidance, positivity, respect, and love. This is what will make it easier for the anxious child to join.

Habit – This last reason seems like the best place to talk about declarative language and age. I want you to know that it is *never* too late to start using declarative language.

It is never too late to start using declarative language.

75

If a child, or adult for that matter, has been exposed primarily to question-asking or directive-based communication their whole life, they need time to get used to a different way of interacting with people. In other words, if individuals have habitually been told what to do or have been socially engaged via question-asking most of the time, their communication skills have likely become reliant on prompts from others to know how and when to initiate, respond to, and join a social exchange.

An important part of any social engagement is spontaneity and independent thought. This is what makes social exchanges meaningful and real. But these are big skills to develop for all communicators! And if an individual has been prompted with directives and questions for a long time, it may take time to reverse that person's reliance on prompts. Both the individual and their communication partners need persistence and patience to form a new communication pattern habit.

Here is an example:

I have been working with Christopher, the young man I previously mentioned, for the past 7 years. When I met him he was 21 years old. His mother, Judy, contacted me because she wanted to help him better express himself and establish deeper communication. At the time, she primarily spoke to him in imperatives (questions and commands) and didn't know if Christopher would respond to this new type of language. As we got started, there were moments where we had to hang in there and have faith. We had to wait, and troubleshoot a lot, as this speaking style was vastly different from what Christopher was used to. But Judy embraced it and began talking to him in a declarative way as much as she could.

It has been exciting to see that as time passed, Christopher's communication changed dramatically. I am happy to say that he now shares much more information with others than he ever did before. His sharing includes what he is thinking about now as well as memories from the past. Judy believes that the memories have always been there, but Christopher didn't have the language skills to share them. He has a unique communication style that he uses to share his memories, but these are authentic memories nonetheless.

Here are examples of memories that I personally observed Christopher share. They are notable not only because of his vivid recollections, but also because they reflect his developing curiosity of the world.

Judy and Christopher often take the train to meet me somewhere in the community. During one visit, Christopher began talking about a sign at the Salem train station that he noticed and liked. In his unique way, he asked why the sign at the train station that day was different than the sign that was there when he visited the Salem train station as a child.

On another day, we were at a museum and stopped to appreciate a painting titled "Athens." Christopher spontaneously made a connection and talked about a vacation their family took to Greece as child. He remembered the name of the cruise line they took and an island they visited, long after his mother had forgotten.

It is amazing to be a part of this growth. Christopher shares these gems more often now, but I feel it is important to remember how quiet he had been for so long.

Here is a recent email from Judy, reflecting on what these changes have meant to her:

Did I tell you about an amazing "memory-sharing" experience I had with Christopher back in May, concerning his memories of a book we used to read to him and how the garden/trees at his house in Canton reminded him of it? If not, I will next time I see you. It felt like a breakthrough kind of thing, as did the three-way Thomas "conversation" we had last time we saw you. Even though these little development steps he takes seem small when I think of the mountain of development he would need to be, say, independent, they mean the WORLD to me. Thank you so much for helping us.

I have one last breathtaking example to share. When Eliza was 3, her family took a vacation where they stayed in a cabin. One night, Eliza had a big tantrum. Her parents could never figure out why and it was upsetting to everyone. Years later, Eliza had the language to explain it! She shared that she had seen a big bug on the wall and had felt frightened. What relief to finally know the reason, and that information, provided by Eliza alone, helped everyone reframe their memories from that night in a positive, understanding way.

Memories are there for your kids too. If this change in speaking style is a big change for the child or adult because they have fallen into the habit of sharing information in response to imperative prompts, hang in there. Stay consistent with your declarative language and have faith that changes can happen, even if it takes a while. Remember, it's never too late for you and your child to break old habits and change the communication style.

Bottom line: If there is one thing you take away from this chapter, I'd like you to take away this: Always give the child the benefit of the doubt when they don't respond to your declarative statement. There is always a good reason, and often it is one of the four above: **processing time**, **attention**, **comprehension**, or **habit**. Wait quietly and observe, giving yourself time to determine the reason. Then move forward with troubleshooting!

Always give the child the benefit of the doubt when they don't respond to your declarative statements.

PART 5

PRACTICE

CHAPTER 12

Practice Sets to Help You Get Comfortable

Declarative language takes practice! Here are a few practice sets for you to hone your skills and become more comfortable with this way of speaking.

Download copies of these practice sets at www.declarativelanguage.com

Practice Set #1: Declarative or Imperative?

Start out by being mindful and noticing when you are using a declarative or an imperative. Once you notice your imperative comments and questions, you can then work to shift or modify them into declarative statements.

For the following 10 pairs, decide which is the imperative and which is its declarative counterpart.

1a. Sit down.

1b. Here is your chair.

2a. What should you be doing?

2b. Let's look and see what your classmates are getting started on.

3a. Your coat is on the floor.

3b. Pick up your coat.

4a. I'm wondering if you heard what I said.

4b. What did I say?

5a. Tell Daddy what you did today.

5b. Let's tell Daddy together what you did today.

6a. I'm ready for the next page when you are.

6b. Turn the page.

7a. What is next?

7b. I'm wondering if you know what to do next.

8a. Your friend looks interested in that toy too.

8b. Give your friend a turn.

9a. What is this a picture of?

9b. I notice something interesting here. I wonder if you know what it's called.

10a. Get the ball.

10b. The balled rolled over there.

Practice Set #2: Changing Imperatives into Declaratives

Change the imperative statements or questions on the next page into declarative statements. Use the words from the word bank below if needed.

Word bank/helpful words to keep in mind

Verbs	Words that Communicate Alternatives and Possibility	Inviting Pronouns	Nouns
think	sometimes	I	idea
notice	perhaps	we	thought
hear	sure	us	opinion
wonder	not sure	let's	preference
decide	maybe		decision
I bet	might		
feel	could		
know	possibly		
don't know			
I see			
wish			
agree			
disagree			
like			
don't like			
hope			
looks			

1. What should you be doing right now?
2. Give me your paper.
3. Pick up those books.
4. What do you need?
5. Buckle your seatbelt.
6. Take a seat.
7. Stop running.
8. Move over.
9. What should you say?
10. Take your turn.

Practice Set #3: Troubleshooting

Imagine that you have made the following declarative statement, but the child did not respond. What are some things you could do or say next to support the child in that moment?

1. All the kids are seated at the table.
2. Let's get started on your homework.
3. I notice your backpack is on the floor.
4. I sure would love some of that popcorn too.
5. I would love to play this game with you.
6. Your friend is waiting for you to take your turn.
7. I think it's your turn to set the table.
8. The cat's dish is empty.
9. The plant looks thirsty.
10. The trash can is overflowing!

Be patient with yourself – declarative language takes practice but is worth it!

PART 6:

TRACKING PROGRESS AND RESEARCH

CHAPTER 13:
How to Recognize Progress

Now comes the important question of how to know whether using declarative language is working or not. The biggest change will be in the communication landscape overall. It will transition from one that has perhaps been negative or consisted of power struggles, to one that is positive, supportive, and understanding. For example, you may feel more patient with your child, because you understand a bit more the fight/flight/freeze response. You have noticed how your child reacts to demands and imperative language in contrast to declarative statements that are more guiding.

You also might find that you are more flexible. You have begun to realize that as you let go and open yourself to more possibilities, and observe the unique responses and contributions of your child, they too are becoming more open and flexible.

The changes start with the adult and then shift to the child. You are modeling in a heartfelt way what you truly want the child to learn: how to be a patient, understanding, communication partner who hears the other person and thoughtfully responds. You have more empathy now because you understand your child better.

The changes start with the adult and then shift to the child. You are modeling in a heartfelt way what you truly want the child to learn: how to be a patient, understanding, communication partner who hears the other person and thoughtfully responds.

Aside from the big picture changes (you feel better, communication is more positive and supportive, you have more positive exchanges and successes overall) here are some smaller moments to watch for.

You will start to notice your child visually reference more. For example, as you make a declarative statement and wait, do you then see them pick their head up and scan the environment, the materials you may be using, or even to look at other people a bit more? You will also see the child take in visual information more often because you are cluing them into what's important in a guiding way. As we mentioned in a previous chapter, this is different from eye contact. They are not looking in a rote way or because you told them to. They are looking to gain needed information. Watch for it!

You will also start to see more active problem solving. This gets exciting! Whereas you may have typically told the child what to do in the past, you are now finding yourself fading back and allowing them to take the lead or take initiative.

A small example might be if something spills. In the past, you may have told the child to clean it up or even to get a paper towel. Now, you find yourself saying instead, *Huh! a spill!* and then waiting quietly. The result is the child then takes the initiative to get a paper towel to clean it up. You had not given them the space to do this in the past, and now that you are, it feels great!

You are seeing them solve problems once you clue them into the fact that one exists or once you have shown them where the problem is. They are solving more problems because you are mindfully giving them more opportunities to do so. Just as you are changing how you communicate, they are changing how they feel and becoming more competent and empowered.

Your child is solving more problems because you are mindfully giving them more opportunities to do so.

You also may start to see the child more actively repair communication breakdowns. Maybe before, you did all the fixing when there was a misunderstanding. You clarified the breakdown or told your child what to say or what to do. Now you are fading back so that they can notice the breakdown and think through how to repair it on their own. You are giving them more active practice in problem solving when it comes to communication, and as a result, they are becoming more independent in their communication skills. Communication isn't perfect—it is as messy as ever! But the difference is that you are not the one responsible for fixing it. You feel more comfortable fading back to allow your child the chance to do this important work.

Your child is also better able to handle setbacks and disappointments because you have become better at helping them access their episodic memory to see the big picture over time. They know that things happen, and it does not have to be the end of the world. You are better at helping them recall what they need to recall, when they need to, without overwhelming them with too much information. You are also patient and kind in these moments, understanding that the meltdown or disappointment is real for them. They feel it more because important memories are not at their fingertips. You feel more patience for their pain and are therefore a better guide to them in the tough moments.

> **Communication isn't perfect – it's as messy as ever! But the difference is that you are not the one responsible for fixing it. You feel more comfortable fading back to allow your child the chance to do this important work.**

You may also start to witness more instances where your child is communicating to share experiences. For example, maybe like Eliza and Christopher, your child is starting to express and share memories more spontaneously. You are hearing more, but you are also patient in providing information. You share memories and information with a future focus. You know it is not about the questions they answer today, but about the memories and information they can share with others tomorrow.

> **You share memories and information with a future focus. You know it is not about the questions a child answers today, but about the memories and information they can share with others tomorrow.**

You act deliberately as you share information and feelings, with the intention of helping them become stronger in their own ability to share experiences with others in the future. You support them as you consider what's to come rather than get stuck on wanting a specific answer in the present. You let go of your need for an immediate answer. As a result, your child chimes into conversations a bit more, either verbally or nonverbally, and memories come out over time.

Your child's vocabulary has grown! You hear them recognizing and talking about feelings a bit more, because you have helped them understand how they feel and what the cues for that feeling may be. And they are starting to use cognitive verbs too! They talk about their thoughts, wishes, ideas, and opinions more freely, and they don't get upset or stuck when their ideas are different from others.

Your child is feeling more comfortable with other opinions in the moment. They can handle different information now in a new way. They don't perceive it as a threat when someone disagrees or thinks differently. This is because you know how to frame the interaction so that it is not about being right or wrong, but about sharing different ideas. Different opinions are interesting and not hard. You model for them and show them how to share space with others who have different ideas. They are now more capable of sharing space with someone who views the world or a situation differently.

Little moments build to big changes. You are noticing more, capitalizing on more moments, understanding what your child needs more, because declarative language has helped you slow down and stay in tune with the feedback your child is providing. You feel more empowered knowing that your child is capable of great things.

Little moments build to big changes.

On the next page is an example tracking sheet with 10 statements that you can use week to week, and month to month, to measure and reflect upon progress related to your observations. Be sure to complete one before you start so you have an accurate picture of your baseline attitudes and perceptions in these areas.

Progress Tracking Sheet

Date:	Not True	Somewhat True	Very True!
I felt patient with my child this week.			
I noticed my child visually reference people or the environment this week.			
I noticed my child problem solve this week.			
I noticed my child use an important memory, with guidance, this week.			
I noticed my child share memories this week.			
I was better at reading my child's cues this week.			
I felt as though I understood my child better this week.			
My child noticed and repaired communication breakdowns this week.			
My child was open to trying something new this week.			
I felt confident guiding my child to try something new or to think in a different way this week.			

Download a copy of this progress tracking sheet at www.declarativelanguage.com

CHAPTER 14:
The Declarative Language Pilot Project

Unfortunately (or fortunately if you view this as an opportunity) there is little information available right now about the use of declarative language as a strong tool for kids with social learning challenges. For those of us who use it every day, however, we have no doubt of its efficacy and power. The door is wide open for clinicians and researchers to explore and validate this speaking style together.

There are now several studies on the effectiveness of Relationship Development Intervention (RDI) as a therapeutic approach for kids with Autism Spectrum Disorder. On the RDI Connect website, you will see a list of studies conducted by Dr. Jessica Hobson, Dr. Steven E. Gutstein, Dr. Nicole Beurkens, and more. As I mentioned in Chapter 1, I first learned of declarative language when training to be an RDI Consultant. Declarative language is an essential tool and strategy used in RDI, and is taught to parents engaged in this treatment approach. RDI parents all over the world can attest to its power and how this speaking style has helped to make positive changes in their relationship with their child.

RDI parents all over the world can attest to how this speaking style has helped to make positive changes in their relationship with their child.

Declarative Language Handbook

In an effort to contribute personal data, I created my own "Declarative Language Pilot Project" in 2017. I began the project shortly after leading a presentation on declarative language as part of the Burr Family Conference at the Cotting School in Lexington, MA. In this presentation, I included basic information on declarative language such as what it was, along with video clips to illustrate its use. These video clips included my own children as well as clients I've discussed throughout this book.

Wanting to do more, I realized that this presentation was the perfect opportunity to engage interested parents in a pilot project. I'm not a formal researcher, but I do love to analyze findings, spot patterns and use math in my work. I was determined to do my part as best I could with the resources I had. So at the end of the training, I invited parents who were interested in being part of a pilot project that would assess the impact of declarative language to reach out to me.

Three moms connected with me right away, and we started our project two months later. Interestingly, each of these mothers had a teenage son who had already been receiving special education services throughout most of his life. These women had been part of their son's therapy for many years, yet the idea of declarative language was new to them, and something they were eager to learn more about.

Here are excerpts from the emails I received following my initial presentation:

I especially enjoyed the two video clips of Christopher, from making pillows to talking about the advertisement that had changed! Seeing such progress in an older child/young adult was really moving for me.

I loved what you had to say and put declarative language to use as soon as I got home. It was so great I have to share.... It has been my concern and complaint for years that his whole life people have told my son what to do so that he won't answer a question or waits for instruction. He doesn't know how to advocate for himself or hold a conversation. It wasn't a miracle every time I used it, but it was enough that I was blown away when it worked more than once. We actually had a conversation that wasn't only about the movies he loves. Thank you.

I've been mindful to speak using declarative language. It really is quite powerful!

And so, we began! I started by having the women and their sons come to my office to record baseline videos observing their natural interaction style. I also had them complete a baseline questionnaire in which they shared their impressions of current communication with their sons, as well as their own knowledge and feelings of competence with using declarative language. Please see the Appendix for a copy of this questionnaire.

We then used video conferencing to meet every two to three weeks over the course of five months, for a total of seven training sessions. Each session consisted of a review of what had been previously learned, introduction of a new topic or a new use for declarative language, video clips of the moms and sons together to illustrate each idea, assignment of homework, and then a plan for our next date. We would also share highlights from each of the moms' videos and any reasons for celebration.

This pilot program provided an incredibly valuable and supportive learning environment for myself and these women. They improved their skill and comfort in declarative language use, and I learned how to best teach it in a more formal way.

At the end of our time, the moms completed a final questionnaire to share overall impressions plus details about their personal growth and returned to my office where I recorded a final video to formally capture and document changes in their communication style. They also completed a short reflection questionnaire after each homework assignment week to week. (See Appendix for examples)

Over the seven sessions, teaching concepts unfolded in the following way:
- Declarative vs. Imperative
- Using declarative language to guide appraisal: Is something good enough?
- Waiting quietly so kids can make discoveries
- Communication: Sharing experiences, being present, establishing a joint focus of attention
- Communication: Breakdowns and repairs
- Communication: Taking perspective
- Wrap up and Review

In addition, strategies that were emphasized throughout including pacing (waiting quietly), troubleshooting tips ("scaffolding"), and slowing down.

Here are a few powerful quotes from the final questionnaire:

What do you feel you gained as a parent from participation in this project? Please be as specific as possible.

Parent 1: As a parent I gained a way to communicate with my child in a manner that is less forceful and demanding allowing us to work more as a team. It gave me the ability to let conversation flow without always directing it.

Parent 2: This course taught me how to live more in the moment – to take time to pause and truly listen to my son. I believe our spontaneous conversations and activities are more connected and meaningful when I implement the strategies and techniques taught in this course. Purposefully speaking in declarative language has made me a kinder and more compassionate person. It certainly gave me insight into how (my son) thinks and feels.

Parent 3: Techniques to prop open the door for prolonged meaningful communication, and patience to wait for opportunities to share experiences, give and gain perspectives, and guide with meaning.

This course taught me how to live more in the moment – to take time to pause and truly listen to my son.

What do you feel your child gained?
Parent 1: My child gained a sense of autonomy and that his opinion counts.

Parent 2: As I continue to focus on using declarative language and pausing with silence on a daily basis, I've noticed my son is sharing his opinions, thoughts and feelings! I've noticed him taking the initiative, and having more confidence to branch out and try a new task, share an idea and engage in reciprocal conversations – even if the topic is non preferred. When I use declarative language, I notice my son's anxiety and perseverative language tends to be less, and he participates more freely without feeling any judgment!

Parent 3: (He) definitely benefited from having one-on-one time carved out of our busy lives to plan, make, and record videos practicing the techniques on a formal basis. Informally, benefited from having a parent who is mindfully structuring and mentally processing the quality (not just quantity) of our communication. Together, both will lead to a renewed focus on parent-child time as well as modeling successful strategies for other family members to employ.

My child gained a sense of autonomy and that his opinion counts.

How have your interactions with your child changed since the beginning of this project?
Parent 1: We have longer conversations.

Parent 2: When I become aware of difficult conversations, I stop and think: Am I using declarative or imperative language? I make a conscientious effort to regroup and practice my declarative language and the outcome is always a better and more meaningful interaction with my son!

Parent 3: Restored my faith and intuition that even the little moments can add up to making a big difference if they are layered in such a way that they support and encourage the growth and development of communication between partners, whether verbal or nonverbal.

Restored my faith and intuition that even the little moments can add up to making a big difference...

In order to quantitatively measure changes, I reviewed all the baseline and final video tapes and captured relevant data related specifically to the language of each mother/son interaction. In these clips, each mother was presented with an activity that comes directly from RDI's assessment, called the RDA or the Relationship Development Assessment. In this activity, the parent and child are given several model card houses and materials (index cards, tape, scissors) to choose from, and then asked to construct their own as a team. This is typically an activity where the child will need some help.

94

Chapter 14: The Declarative Language Pilot Project

I measured language across specific areas for each mother/son interaction. Measurements began five minutes after the introduction of the activity and lasted for two minutes. I chose this middle two minutes of the activity to allow the individuals time to settle in and get acclimated to the expectations of the task. There is much communication that happens in two minutes of time thus this amount of time was chosen as a beginning snapshot from which to measure communicative patterns.

The following items were measured across each two-minute sample, for each mother/son pair:
- Frequency of parent's questions and commands
- Frequency of parent's comments
- Frequency of son's utterances overall (single words, word combinations and sentences)
- Frequency of son's utterances that were:
  1. Related to what their mother had said
     and
  2. More than one word*
- Frequency of son's utterances that were:
  1. Unrelated to what their mother had said
     and
  2. More than one word

*More than one-word utterances were chosen for measurement to ensure the utterance could be easily categorized as related or unrelated to what their mother had said. Examples:

The following utterance was judged to be related:
Mom: "Okay, you've got tape. I see here…to stretch it across."
Son: "It's hard."

While this utterance was judged to be unrelated:
Mom: "I wonder what we should do first."
Son: "How often do I see Natalie?

In order to include another evaluator and judge in this process, my colleague and fellow RDI Consultant, Elisabeth Ramirez, independently reviewed and categorized each utterance from these samples. Items that we agreed upon were tallied.

The following frequencies were collected.

Parent/ Son 1	Parent questions or commands	Parent comments	Son's utterances	Son's related utterances & >1 word	Son's unrelated utterances & >1 word
January	15	9	7	4	0
June	7	23	8	7	0
% change	-53.33	+155.55	+14.28	+75	No change
Increase or Decrease?	Decrease	Increase	Increase	Increase	No change
Desired effect?	Yes	Yes	--	Yes	n/a

Parent/ Son 2	Parent questions or commands	Parent comments	Son's utterances	Son's related utterances & >1 word	Son's unrelated utterances & >1 word
January	17	15	23	6	4
June	6	22	20	10	0
% change	-64.71	+46.66	-13.04	+66.66	-100
Increase or Decrease?	Decrease	Increase	Decrease	Increase	Decrease
Desired effect?	Yes	Yes	--	Yes	Yes

Parent/ Son 3	Parent questions or commands	Parent comments	Son's utterances	Son's related utterances & >1 word	Son's unrelated utterances & >1 word
January	6	20	2	0	0
June	6	20	4	1	0
% change	No change	No change	+100	Unable to measure	No change
Increase or Decrease?	No change	No change	Increase	Increase	No change
Desired effect?	n/a	n/a	--	yes	n/a

To summarize, from January to June, two of the parents decreased question asking and commands and increased declarative statements, while all sons increased in their related utterances. These snapshot findings are positive and reveal one possible way to measure the effectiveness of declarative language.

These snapshot findings are positive and reveal one possible way to measure the effectiveness of declarative language.

It is also important to note that there are many other possible areas to explore in relation to declarative language that were not within the scope of this project yet could yield noteworthy findings. These include more subtle measures of social connection such as changes in the parent's pacing of communication, instances of visual referencing, and the sharing of positive emotions as evidenced through nonverbal communication (e.g., smiles, laughter, etc.). These measures will be especially important for kids who are less verbal or use alternative forms of communication.

It will also be important to explore subtle measures of social connection such as changes in the parent's pacing of communication, instances of visual referencing, and the sharing of positive emotions as evidenced through nonverbal communication (smiles, laughter, etc.).

There is still much to be done to establish that the positive changes I observed are valid and reliable, and that these changes are related to the use of declarative language. I understand my work here is very preliminary and I humbly present this project as one beginning path toward proving the effectiveness of declarative language. I am excited for what is to come, and for declarative language to receive wider awareness and use.

PART 7:
FINAL WORDS

CHAPTER 15:
Where Do We Go From Here?

Here we are at the end. Or should I say at the beginning? There is so much to do moving forward to help the world know there is a better way when it comes to communicating and speaking to individuals with social learning challenges. As you change your own speaking style, remember to set yourself up for success. Start small in manageable contexts and increase your use of declarative language as you get comfortable and see the difference it can make.

As you change your own speaking style, remember to set yourself up for success.

When sharing information or leading a training on declarative language, I often hear people say, "It sounds great but that will never work with my child/my student, etc." To that person, I say that if you think it won't work, you are probably right, because for declarative language to work, we must approach kids with a positive mindset. If you are negative or skeptical, that is the message the child will receive.

Declarative language is open and supportive, and assumes the student is doing the best they can. It comes with the understanding that a child may be using a negative communication style because that is what life has given them. You give what you get.

Declarative language is open and supportive and assumes the student is doing the best that they can.

To skeptical people I also say: it's not a one-shot deal. We are not asking for the student to do what we want them to do in just one particular instance, and from that conclude declarative language either works or it doesn't. No. We are going for a shift in the entire communicative landscape that a child is used to. We are there to teach them over time that there is a different way. We are working to shift a typically negative or demand-based pattern of communication to a positive one. But these things take time.

We are going for a shift in the entire communicative landscape that a child is used to. We are there to teach them over time that there is a different way.

We cannot expect to make one declarative comment and for the dynamic to immediately shift. This is not a quick fix. We must hang in there and show kids we mean it. We want them to believe that we have changed our style and mindset to one that views them in a positive light. Keep in mind that *anything* that matters takes time and effort. Think about going to the moon! We are working to change the tide for these students. To help them open themselves up to the world and to learning. To help them trust. To help them lower their defenses. We start small because that is the only way to do it – one exchange at a time. And these small moments will build up and create positive momentum.

We start small because that is the only way to do it – one exchange at a time.

So, in day to day life, you will start one interaction at a time. And start at a place that keeps you feeling increasingly more comfortable and confident with your change in speaking style. In the long term, you will be changing the dynamic of communication with your child or student from negative to positive.

I want readers to remember Christopher as an illustration of this, but also as evidence that it is never too late to introduce declarative language. I met him at age 21, and within two years he was sharing some memories, and by age 26 these were coming out more and more. It is never too late to create this experience-sharing environment, but it takes commitment and belief that communication can be better. And it starts with you!

I absolutely acknowledge that we need research for declarative language to stick. I'd love to find ways to broadcast this approach and its effectiveness to a wider audience, so that it becomes a strategy that is consistently taught to those who will be educating kids with social learning challenges – including teachers, therapists, and parents. In order to get to this place, research is needed so that declarative language makes it into textbooks and classroom discussions automatically.

In my experience, I think the most powerful measures of progress will be via parent perception and in the ways a child's communication changes over time. I also think that progress would have to be measured over the course of months or years, because, as I've said, it takes time to shift a communicative landscape.

I would love any help designing a study to duplicate my beginning findings or to think through a different way to measure the positive results of declarative language. If you are a researcher who has ideas and this interests you, please contact me.

Declarative language is a powerful, but underused strategy. It doesn't have to be. What we say and how we say it matters. Help me change the world for kids and adults with social learning challenges by spreading this important message.

APPENDIX

To follow are the questionnaires I used in my 2017 Declarative Language Pilot Project:

1. Baseline Caregiver Questionnaire
2. Example Video Reflection Worksheet (Worksheet 5 – Communication Breakdowns and Repairs)
3. Final Caregiver Questionnaire

Declarative Language Handbook

1. **Declarative Language Pilot Project – Baseline Caregiver Questionnaire**

Today's Date:
Child's Name: **Child's DOB:**
Person completing this form: **Relationship to child:**

1. On a scale of 1-5, where 1 = Novice and 5 = Proficient, how comfortable do you feel with your own use of declarative language? Please circle:

1	2	3	4	5
Novice				Proficient

2. What do you hope to gain from participation in this project?

Please circle the number that best applies to each statement, where *1=Rarely* and *3=Often:*

	Rarely	Sometimes	Often
3. My child spontaneously initiates communication with me.	1	2	3
4. I feel emotionally close to my child.	1	2	3
5. My child and I laugh together.	1	2	3
6. I prompt my child to do things.	1	2	3
7. I prompt my child to answer questions.	1	2	3
8. My child looks at me when communicating.	1	2	3
9. My child uses language to meet his/her immediate needs.	1	2	3
10. My child uses language to share his/her memories, opinions, ideas and observations.	1	2	3
11. I have back and forth exchanges with my child where I don't prompt him/her.	1	2	3

12. Please share an anecdote or example of a typical communicative exchange with your child.

Thank you for your responses!

Appendix

2. Declarative Language Pilot Project
Video Reflections Worksheet 5 – Communication Breakdowns and Repairs

Today's Date:
Child's Name: Child's DOB:
Person completing this form: Relationship to child:

1. What activity did you choose to do with your child?

2. What were some of the communication breakdowns that you noticed during this activity?

Upon review of the clip, what did you notice about the interaction?	Rarely	Sometimes			Often
3. I asked my child questions.	1	2	3	4	5
4. I made comments.	1	2	3	4	5
5. I shared my feelings, memories, opinions and experiences.	1	2	3	4	5
6. I used first person pronouns such as *I, we, us, our,* and *let's.*	1	2	3	4	5
7. I felt that we established and maintained a joint focus of attention.	1	2	3	4	5
8. I was present in the moment.	1	2	3	4	5
9. I recognized the reason for communication breakdowns.	1	2	3	4	5
10. I named the reason for communication breakdowns using declarative language.	1	2	3	4	5
11. After I commented upon the breakdown, I quietly waited to allow time for my child to spontaneously make a repair.	1	2	3	4	5
12. I guided my child on how to make a repair when needed.	1	2	3	4	5
13. I am kind to myself. I use positive self-talk while I learn something new.	1	2	3	4	5

14. What did you like about this clip?

15. What things did you notice that you might do differently next time?

16. Were there any incidental communication breakdown/communicative repair opportunities that you found yourself embracing in the moment since our last training?

17. Any questions for Linda?

Declarative Language Handbook

3. **Declarative Language Pilot Project – Final Caregiver Questionnaire**
Part 1 - Reflections

Today's Date:
Child's Name: **Child's DOB:**
Person completing this form: **Relationship to child:**

1. On a scale of 1-5, where 1 = Novice and 5 = Proficient, how comfortable do you feel with your own use of declarative language? Please circle:

1	2	3	4	5
Novice				Proficient

2. What do you feel you gained as a parent from participation in this project? Please be as specific as possible.

3. What do you feel your child gained?

4. How have your interactions with your child changed since the beginning of this project?

Please circle the number that best applies to each statement, where *1=Rarely* and *3=Often:*

	Rarely	Sometimes	Often
5. My child spontaneously initiates communication with me.	1	2	3
6. I feel emotionally close to my child.	1	2	3
7. My child and I laugh together.	1	2	3
8. I prompt my child to do things.	1	2	3
9. I prompt my child to answer questions.	1	2	3
10. My child looks at me when communicating.	1	2	3
11. My child uses language to meet his/her immediate needs.	1	2	3
12. My child uses language to share his/her memories, opinions, ideas and observations.	1	2	3
13. I have back and forth exchanges with my child where I don't prompt him/her.	1	2	3

14. Please share an anecdote or example of a recent communicative exchange with your child.

106

Appendix

Part 2 – Feedback for Linda - Please rate and provide any comments

How helpful was each part of our trainings?	Not helpful	Somewhat helpful			Very helpful
Check-in: reflections, discussion, questions	1	2	3	4	5
Comments, feedback or ideas to make this better?					
Review of homework videos	1	2	3	4	5
Comments, feedback or ideas to make this better?					
Presentation of new concepts					
Definition/Explanation of Idea	1	2	3	4	5
Mechanics	1	2	3	4	5
Video examples	1	2	3	4	5
Comments, feedback or ideas to make this better?					
Homework Assignment	1	2	3	4	5
Comments, feedback or ideas to make this better?					

Declarative Language Handbook

How valuable did you find each concept?	Not valuable	Somewhat valuable			Very valuable
Training 1: Declarative vs. Imperative *Comments, feedback or ideas to make this better?*	1	2	3	4	5
Training 2: Appraisal *Comments, feedback or ideas to make this better?*	1	2	3	4	5
Training 3: Discoveries *Comments, feedback or ideas to make this better?*	1	2	3	4	5
Training 4: Experience Sharing *Comments, feedback or ideas to make this better?*	1	2	3	4	5
Training 5: Breakdowns and Repairs *Comments, feedback or ideas to make this better?*	1	2	3	4	5
Training 6: Taking Perspective *Comments, feedback or ideas to make this better?*	1	2	3	4	5
Training 7: Wrap-up and review *Comments, feedback or ideas to make this better?*	1	2	3	4	5

Appendix

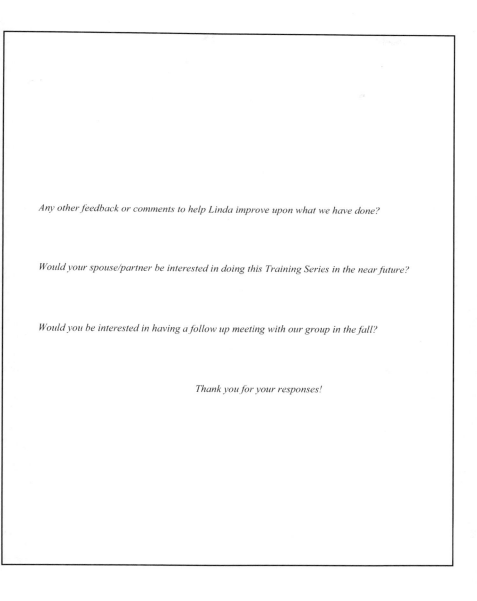

Any other feedback or comments to help Linda improve upon what we have done?

Would your spouse/partner be interested in doing this Training Series in the near future?

Would you be interested in having a follow up meeting with our group in the fall?

Thank you for your responses!

BIBLIOGRAPHY

Braaten, E. & Willoughby, B. (2014). *Bright kids who can't keep up.* New York, NY: The Guilford Press.

Brown, B. (2010). *The gifts of imperfection: Let go of who you think you're supposed to be and embrace who you are.* Center City, MN: Hazelden Publishing.

Cook, B. & Garnett, M. (2018). *Spectrum women.* London: Jessica Kingsley Publishers.

Cook, J. (2008). *Don't be afraid to drop!* Chattanooga, TN: National Center for Youth Issues.

Deak, J. (2010). *Your fantastic, elastic brain: Stretch it, shape it.* Naperville, IL: Little Pickle Press.

Dweck, C.S. (2007). *Mindset: The new psychology of success.* New York, NY: Ballantine Books.

Fredrickson, B.L. (2004). The broaden-and-build theory of positive emotions. *Philosophical Transactions of the Royal Society B: Biological Sciences.* 359(1449): 1367–1378.

Garland, E.L., Fredrickson, B., Kring, A.M., Johnson, D.P., Meyer, P.S., & Penn, D.L. (2010). Upward spirals of positive emotions counter downward spirals of negativity: Insights from the broaden-and-build theory and affective neuroscience on the treatment of emotion dysfunctions and deficits in psychopathology. *Clinical Psychology Review,* 30(7), 849-64.

Grandin, T. & Panek, R. (2013). *The Autistic brain: Thinking across the spectrum.* New York, NY: Houghton Mifflin Harcourt Publishing.

Greene, R. (2016). *Lost and found: Helping behaviorally challenging students (and while you're at it, all the others).* San Francisco, CA: Jossey-Bass.

Greene, R. (2008). *Lost at school: Why our kids with behavioral challenges are falling through the cracks and how we can help them.* New York, NY: Scribner.

Groden, J., Kantor, A, Woodard, C & Lipsitt, L. (2011). *How everyone on the Autism Spectrum, young and old, can ...:Become resilient, be more optimistic, enjoy humor, be kind, and increase self-efficacy – A positive psychology approach.* London: Jessica Kingsley Publishers.

Gutstein, S. E. (2009). Empowering families through Relationship Development Intervention®: an important part of the biopsychosocial management of autism spectrum disorders. *Annals of Clinical Psychiatry,* 21(3), 174-82.

Gutstein, S.E. (2004). Relationship Development Intervention®: Developing a treatment program to address the unique social and emotional deficits in Autism Spectrum Disorder. *Autism Spectrum Quarterly,* Winter, 8-12.

Gutstein, S.E. (2004). The effectiveness of Relationship Development Intervention® on remediating core deficits of autism-spectrum children. *Journal of Developmental and Behavioral Pediatrics,* 25(5), 275.

Gutstein, S. E. (2009). *The RDI book: Forging new pathways for Autism, Asperger's and PDD with the Relationship Development Intervention ® Program.* Houston, TX: Connections Center Publishing.

Gutstein, S. E., Burgess, A. F., & Montfort, K. (2007). Evaluation of the Relationship Development Intervention® Program. *Autism: The International Journal of Research and Practice,* 11(5), 397-411.

Gutstein, S. E. (2007). *Relationship Development Intervention® (RDI®) Program and education.* Houston, TX: Connections Center Publishing.

Hobson, J. A., Hobson, P., Gutstein, S., Ballarani, A., Bargiota, K. (2008). Caregiver-child relatedness in autism, what changes with intervention? Poster presented at the meeting of the *International Meeting for Autism Research.*

Hobson, J. A., Tarver, L., Beurkens, N., & Hobson, R. P. (2016). The relation between severity of Autism and caregiver-child interaction: A study in the context of Relationship Development Intervention. *Journal of Abnormal Child Psychology.* 44(4), 745-55.

Bibliography

Kedar, I. (2012). *Ido in Autismland: Climbing out of Autism's silent prison*. Sharon Kedar.

Keller, G. (2013). *The ONE thing: The surprisingly simple truth behind extraordinary results*. Austin, TX: Bard Press.

Kim, C. (2014). *Nerdy, shy and socially inappropriate: A user guide to an Asperger life*. London: Jessica Kingsley Publishers.

Jones, C. (1994). *Mistakes that worked: 40 familiar inventions & how they came to be*. New York, NY: Delacorte Books for Young Readers.

Kuypers, L. (2011). *The Zones of Regulation: A curriculum designed to foster self-regulation and emotional control*. Santa Clara, CA: Think Social Publishing, Inc.

Murphy, L.K. (2010). Episodic memory, experience sharing, and children with ASD. *Autism Spectrum Quarterly*, Fall, 15-16.

Murphy, L.K. (2012). Thinking beyond eye contact. *Autism Spectrum Quarterly*, Winter, 15-16.

Murphy, L.K. (2010). The critical importance of declarative language input for children with ASD. *Autism Spectrum Quarterly*, Winter, 8-10.

Murphy, L.K. (2019). The importance of sharing personal memories to make language meaningful. *Autism Asperger's Digest*, February – April, 33-35.

Murphy, L.K. (2018). What we say and how we say it matters. *Autism Asperger's Digest,* August – October, 32-33.

Larkin, F., Guerin, S., Hobson, J. A., & Gutstein, S. E. (2015). The relationship development assessment – research version: Preliminary validation of a clinical tool and coding schemes to measure parent-child interaction in autism. *Clinical Child Psychology and Psychiatry,* 20(2), 239-60.

Parish, P. (2013). *Amelia Bedelia.* Broadway, NY: Greenwillow Books.

Prizant, B. M. (2010). Respect begins with language: Part I. *Autism Spectrum Quarterly,* Summer, 26-28.

Prizant, B. M. (2010). Respect begins with language: Part II. *Autism Spectrum Quarterly,* Fall, 29-33.

Prizant, B. M. (2011). The use and misuse of evidence-based practice: Implications for persons with ASD. *Autism Spectrum Quarterly,* Fall, 43-49.

Prizant, B. M. (2009). Treatment options and parent choice: Is ABA the only way? Part II. *Autism Spectrum Quarterly,* Spring, 28-32.

Prizant, B. M., and Laurent, A.C. (2011). Behavior is not the issue: An emotional regulation perspective on problem behavior: Part I. *Autism Spectrum Quarterly,* Spring, 28-30.

Bibliography

Prizant, B. M., and Laurent, A.C. (2011) Behavior is not the issue: An emotional regulation perspective on Problem Behavior: Part II. *Autism Spectrum Quarterly,* Summer, 34-37.

Saltzberg, B. (2010). *Beautiful oops!* New York, NY: Workman Publishing Company.

Siegel, D. (2015). *Brainstorm: The power and purpose of the teenage brain.* New York, NY: Tarcher-Perigee.

Siegel, D. (2014). *Parenting from the inside out: How a deeper self-understanding can help you raise children who thrive.* New York, NY: Jeremy P. Tarcher/Penguin.

Siegel, D. (2012). *The developing mind: How relationships and the brain interact to shape who we are.* New York, NY: The Guildford Press.

Siegel, D. & Bryson, T.P. (2012). *The whole-brain child: 12 revolutionary strategies to nurture your child's developing mind.* New York, NY: Bantam.

Spires, A. (2014). *The most magnificent thing.* Toronto: Kids Can Press.

Winner, M.G. (2000). *Inside out: What makes a person with social cognitive deficits tick?* Santa Clara, CA: Think Social Publishing, Inc.

Winner, M.G. (2006). *Social Behavior Mapping: Introducing the social emotional chain reaction.* Santa Clara, CA: Think Social Publishing, Inc.

Winner, M.G., & Murphy L.K. (2016). *Social thinking and me.* Santa Clara, CA: Think Social Publishing, Inc.

Winner, M.G. (2007). *Thinking about you. Thinking about me.* Santa Clara, CA: Think Social Publishing, Inc.

INDEX

Index

Aboard Cabrillo's Galleon

To Ed and Gloria,

Enjoy this glimpse of early California.

Love,
Chris